Ina M...

ARTHRITIS IS
YOUR SUFFERING
REALLY NECESSARY?

Overcoming Common Problems

Overcoming Common Problems

ARTHRITIS IS
YOUR SUFFERING
REALLY NECESSARY?

Dr William Fox
M.B., M.R.C.S.

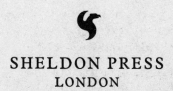

SHELDON PRESS
LONDON

First published in Great Britain in 1981 by
Robert Hale Limited, London

First published in paperback in Great Britain in 1982 by
Sheldon Press, SPCK,
Marylebone Road, London, NW1 4DU

British Library Cataloguing in Publication Data

Fox, William W.
　　Arthritis: is your suffering really necessary?
　　1. Rheumatism　　2. Arthritis
　　I. Title
　　616.7′2′　　　RC927

　　ISBN 0–85969–372–4

Printed in Great Britain by
Richard Clay (The Chaucer Press) Ltd,
Bungay, Suffolk

Contents

To my dear wife Sybia
who actually enjoyed deciphering,
anotating and typing my somewhat
illegible script

Preface

MEDICAL PRIDE AND SCIENTIFIC PREJUDICE
D. L. J. Freed, MD
Lecturer in Immunology
Manchester University

A few years ago I broke my leg in a motorcycle accident. The fracture was severe and complicated, and one of the nerves in my leg was cut by a sharp fragment of bone. The bone was efficiently set in hospital, the nerve gradually recovered, and today I am almost as good as new. But I cannot think back to my weeks in hospital without feelings of horror and anger, because although I suffered severe pain for many months, I was not given effective pain-killing drugs for longer than three days. When I tried to tell the young doctors and nurses about my agony, I was frankly disbelieved, accused of becoming addicted. So tension and suspicion poisoned the relationship when there should have been only trust. Why was I disbelieved? Because the traditional hospital teaching states that severe pain after a fracture lasts for forty-eight hours. I was in fact given morphine for one day after that deadline, but perhaps that was because I too am a doctor.

Years later a patient came to see me complaining of attacks of pins and needles in hands and feet, together with shortness of temper and depression. I am a specialist in allergy, and he arrived at my clinic because his attacks were brought on (he claimed) by eating certain foodstuffs, par-

ticularly monosodium glutamate. He had already been seen
by a number of other doctors, who examined him carefully
(he too was a doctor), performed the relevant tests and
found nothing wrong. So they finally told him that his
symptoms were imaginary, leaving him not only ill but
humiliated and angry.

My own experience had taught me some humility, so I
told him that, although I had never heard of this kind of
thing before, I was prepared to believe that his illness was
genuine and physical and would investigate it seriously.
Instead of repeating the tests he had already had, I asked
him to attend on a day when he felt completely well. I
measured his nerve-conductance every fifteen minutes and
took blood-samples repeatedly throughout that afternoon.
After the first half-hour I persuaded him to eat a cooked
pork pie containing monosodium glutamate (he was most
reluctant as he knew it would make him ill). As he had
predicted, his symptoms began after ten minutes, together
with changes in the nerve-conductances. When the blood-
tests results came back, it transpired that he had also had
complement activation (a sign of acute systemic inflammation) at the same moment. On other occasions we repeated
the performance but without the pork pie 'challenge'—
neither the symptoms nor the neurological or biochemical
changes occurred. So the story had a happy ending, not
because I cured him (I could not) but because I believed him
and was able to provide objective evidence of his truthful-
ness.

So why had the other doctors not believed him? I can
think of three reasons. The story was unusual (in fact,
unique); they could not think of a plausible theory to
explain it on a physical basis; and they *could* think of a
plausible theory to explain it on a mental basis—i.e. he was
either a hypochondriac or hysterical or malingering. And
they preferred to believe the latter explanation in spite of his
apparent sincerity and intelligence. But they were wrong.
They had excluded all the diseases that they knew about—
indeed all diseases that were known—but had not excluded
diseases that they did not know about, including (as it
turned out) a process that at the time had not been dis-

covered. What they *should* have said to him was, "We do not know the cause of your symptoms."

Doctors do not like to admit to patients—or indeed to themselves—that they are not all-knowing and all-wise. We are trained to appear confident even if we are not. If faced with a bizarre case that does not fit our preconceptions, we are tempted to ignore or dismiss the 'wrong' bits—to fit the patient's story into our prejudices instead of *vice versa*. But this is unscientific, foolish and wrong. Prejudice is the enemy of truth, in medicine as in all other areas. Doctors must certainly maintain a high degree of scepticism, not believing anything without good evidence, but on the other hand we must also be open-minded. Many doctors believe that 'Science' is a body of textbook knowledge, a mass of facts to be swallowed and remembered, but this is not true. Science is an attitude of mind, a disciplined curiosity, highly sceptical but always aware that anything is possible.

The author of this book is a conventionally trained British doctor. Like many other doctors, he became dissatisfied with his training as over the years he found himself faced with problems for which the textbooks had no answers. So, not knowing what to expect, he started listening more carefully to what patients said, discarding nothing, prepared to believe that it was all true. And even though at first some of the things they said made no sense to him, gradually an overall picture began to emerge. He was able to formulate theories, then test them, modify them in the light of his experiments, then test them again. Modestly, he makes no claim to being a 'scientist', yet that is exactly what he is. As a fellow scientist I salute him and treat his views with utmost respect. If other 'experts' have failed to do so, that is a criticism of them, not of him.

Introduction

Fifty years ago we could diagnose advanced cancer, but we still cannot cure it. Fifty years ago we could diagnose arthritis, but we still cannot cure it. It is not even properly understood.

There is reasonable hope of solving the cancer problem because we have traced its origin back to the starting-point—the abnormal behaviour of the body cells which represent the basic bricks of the human body. I believe we have now realized that the discovery of a cancer in any one area of the body is just a local manifestation of a disease-process which really affects the whole body.

We also know that cancers vary in their severity; some develop very slowly whilst others are very rapid. The apparent success or failure of operations and other forms of treatment, such as deep X-rays or cobalt radiation, depends very much on the development-rate of the cancer. Some forms of blood cancer are now treated with drugs, which attack what is believed to be the cancer-forming process, based on precise scientific investigation, and are producing much more hopeful results. This promising stage has been reached because of the incessant demand to diagnose the cancer condition in its very early stages. This demand was based on an assumption that, if only we could get the cases early enough, surgery would cure it. Although we have now found this not to be wholly true, it has enabled us to study the disease both clinically and scientifically at a much earlier stage than an obvious lump, thus giving us a greater and more detailed understanding of its behaviour, development, and how to deal with it. In certain types of cancer, particularly in the bowel, even though a complete cure cannot be guaranteed by operation, considerable numbers of people are enabled to live happy and much longer lives as a result of the surgeon's skill. In these cases, the earlier the diagnosis is made the better are the results. It is estimated that some of these cancers may take two to four years to reach a size that would cause recognizable symptoms, and it may be even longer. On the basis of such a (not unreasonable) hypothesis, survival for five or more years is to be expected and frequently happens.

If we compare dry rot in the house with cancer in the body, we may get a clearer idea of the problem. Before the dry-rot fungus creeps in between the bricks of the wall, or causes cracks in the skirting-board, it has been growing from seed or roots in the earth on which the foundations of the house are laid. It can take years for it to develop and bypass the damp-course before it gets through to the skirting-board, floors and bricks. As in cancer, you can eradicate all the fungus you can see, together with rotten wood, bricks and damp-course. If you now rebuild, it would take at least the same number of years for the fungus to reappear. In dry-rot you can, however, kill the fungus seeds and roots with chemicals, so that there is, practically speaking, no likelihood of its return. When we have discovered what causes the cancer cell to develop, we shall most probably find a drug to eliminate it, just as they can now do with the dry-rot fungus. This would then allow normal healthy tissues to develop.

I want to repeat that all this progress and the promise for the future have been achieved because we can recognize cancer in its relatively early development.

What now of arthritis?

Fifty years ago we described many forms of this disease,

such as spondylitis, osteo-arthritis, rheumatoid arthritis. We still talk about them as different diseases, and their diagnosis rests on X-ray evidence. The standard attitude in rheumatology is that, if there is no X-ray evidence of arthritis, then you have not got it. How like the attitude to cancer fifty years ago! If you had not got a lump to feel or an X-ray picture to show, then they could not diagnose cancer. How different today—they have detailed symptoms which might lead to a suspicion of cancer, and then advanced technology to pursue the investigation.

The rheumatologists do not seem to have realized that there is a parallel in these two types of disease. To understand arthritis, you must be able to recognize its onset long before the X-rays show damage to the joints. By this time it is like being able to feel a cancer with your hand or finding dry-rot in the skirting-board.

I have spent my life trying to piece together the evidence which would demonstrate how arthritis first develops. As far back as 1950 I wrote a treatise on the chronic rheumatic diseases. In it, I pointed out the folly of classifying these diseases on X-ray evidence. I explained that this classification was based on long-established disease and that it laid emphasis on the differences rather than the similarities of the differing types. Such an attitude would, therefore, work against the idea that they may be variations of the same basic disease which must have started long before there was enough damage of the joints to be visible on X-ray pictures.

My researches have pointed unerringly to the fact that all forms of arthritis start as an inflammatory condition of the soft tissues, what we call connective tissue, ligaments and tendons near the joints. Only later are the joints affected. In other words, they probably start as the common rheumatic complaints of all ages which most people have at some time during their lives. In childhood it could be 'growing pains', later on backache, fibrositis, lumbago or even sprains of the arm or leg. You will find all this clearly explained in the book. Unhappily the rheumatology mind is still focused on the arthritic joints, just as the surgical mind fifty years ago was concentrated on the actual cancer growth.

I have wondered for a long time why it is so difficult to get any new idea even looked at, never mind accepted, by the medical profession, and I believe the answer lies in (1) the method of education and training of doctors, and (2) the unique position they hold in society.

From the age of about fifteen, the prospective doctor studies chemistry, physics and biology at school, in preparation for the medical course.

In the university, medical scientific subjects including anatomy are taught. On to the hospitals, where diseases are studied. Possibly the only 'normal' subject that is studied is obstetrics, but there again it is abnormal aspects which are detailed.

Theoretically on qualification the doctors should be able to diagnose and treat every known disease. By the time apprenticeship is served, about another two years, the doctors are getting on for twenty-five years old. What do they know about people and normality? What do they know of the Humanities and the Arts? They have had precious little time for anything outside their training. It is only when they are launched on the public that they are ever likely to learn what real life is all about. It is certainly not illness, that is the last thing people want, but the only subject most doctors know.

The good doctor is the one who is aware of this incongruity and tries to learn what life is all about. To do this requires humility, and that, most unfortunately, is not an outstanding characteristic of the profession. To understand why this is so, we must consider the unique position doctors occupy in society.

The medical profession is remarkable in that its work is very rarely criticized, either as a body or as individuals. This is because we practise a subject which is not understood by the lay person and which is in marked contrast to the Arts, the other professions and business, where failure to reach standards or to produce results can be recognized and criticized.

During the training-period—that is, from a student up to senior registrar stage, advice and criticism is available and is wisely given, but once a doctor reaches the specialist grade or goes into general practice, he is unlikely to be subjected to further criticism. For obvious reasons, a consultant would never be criticized by those below him, and a general practitioner works more or less in isolation.

This state of affairs is particularly bad for the general practitioner, who is mostly on his own soon after qualification and, as I shall demonstrate, not well equipped for his job. The fact that errors are not subject to criticism is bad enough, but, unfortunately, the absence of criticism throughout the practising period of a GP or a specialist inevitably tends to produce a sense of security in their ability which may not be really justified. However valid criticism may be, it is never really popular with the recipients, even though they, like artists, actors and writers, may be used to it. I realize, therefore, that it is even less acceptable to members of the medical profession, who have never really been subjected to precise criticism.

I do not want to give the impression that I see nothing good in medical practice. This is far from the truth. I respect very greatly the technical achievements in all the specialist branches; I am aware that most GPs carry on their practices as efficiently and conscientiously as their knowledge and circumstances will allow. No matter how good the present standards are thought to be, there is considerable room for further improvement. There is a vast area of chronic ill health which is not understood by the profession and for which the doctors can do little except use pain-relievers, tranquillizers and physical medicine, either after or before exhaustive and expensive investigations have failed to make the patients' symptoms fit into any recognizable disease-pattern.

If the doctors do not know the cause of the patients' symptoms, how can they possibly expect to treat them successfully? The answer is that they cannot, but they have no sense of guilt or failure about it because of their medical education. This education has produced qualified practitioners who think they know all that is required of them to practise successfully and that any further progress in diagnosis and treatment will be achieved by the scientific pursuit of research in the laboratories and hospitals.

The persistence of ill health destroys the quality of people's lives. I believe that it is more important, more desirable and indeed more moral to give priority to this consideration than to make our prime objective the prolongation of a life whose quality has been eroded by pain, suffering and incurable disease.

The art and science of medicine should be concerned primarily with the healing of the sick. That should be the only reason for our existence—that and the trust that patients must perforce place in us. To merit this trust, the profession must constantly subject their own efforts to self-criticism and ask why, with so much 'progress', there is so much ill health.

What we were all taught as medical students was about diseases, how to diagnose and treat them. What I began to learn as a practising doctor for fifty years was about people, their anxieties and so many of their complaints which did not appear in medical textbooks or in the hospital wards. As soon as I met a case which I did not understand simply because it had not been taught, I realized there was no dialogue between the patient and me. I was listening to symptoms which could not be translated into known disease and which therefore could not be properly treated.

I was very surprised and shocked that with such inadequate knowledge I must accept the responsibility of so much ill health. In trying to bring some understanding into this vast area, I developed a practical approach to the treatment of many common problems in general practice and a much greater understanding of the widespread rheumatic diseases and allied conditions.

The medical profession will find in this book an explanation of so much which is not understood, such as tension, strain, migraine and psychosomatic or neurotic illnesses. The lay public will very soon recognize many of their symptoms with a rational explanation for them. I can see no harm coming from this. On the contrary, it should increase understanding on both sides, and this can lead only to improved diagnosis and treatment.

During all the fifty years I have worked as a general practitioner and as a specialist in the rheumatic diseases, it had never once occurred to me that I would wish to denigrate my colleagues. All that I had ever hoped to do was to make a contribution towards the knowledge and understanding of so much disease for which we can do so little. What I have discovered is fully detailed in this book. What I have to say is as much the concern of the public as it is of the medical profession.

1

Why I Wrote this Book

As far back as I can remember, I was always going to be a doctor. In spite of my name being Fox, I was saddled with the Christian name of Woolfe because that was the name of my uncle who was a doctor. 'William' was promoted to my first name and 'Woolfe' relegated to 'W' to save me from the boring remarks of my school 'friends' relating to the menagerie.

Although I had a very marked mathematical and scientific bent, I had to relinquish maths, physics and chemistry for what then corresponded to A levels because of some difficulties with my chemistry master, and studied English, French and German, which became the stepping-stones to Manchester University. These subjects were a most unusual combination for a pre-medical education, but I have since realized how invaluable this cultural education was in forming a more mature attitude to life and a deeper understanding of human nature. I believe this made me a better doctor than would otherwise have been the case.

In this context it is worthwhile reminding ourselves that, in the Churchill era of the war and immediately afterwards, genuine concern for one another and not self-interest was at its peak. Most public discussions came not only from the mind but also from the heart. For example, educational and philosophic opinions were expressed that, in order to promote better understanding between the sciences and the arts, which are there to serve mankind, those concerned with the arts should have a grounding in the sciences, whilst those concerned with science should have a grounding in the arts. I was the involuntary guinea-pig of this philosophy long before that, in 1921.

When I qualified as a doctor, my brain was crammed full of knowledge of the human body, its anatomy, how it functioned, all the diseases that could afflict it, how to diagnose and treat them. I was the finished product of medical training and education, ready and willing to deal with all the problems of ill health of anyone who wished to consult me!

I spent the first two years gaining experience. Some of the time I worked as a house surgeon and house physician in various hospitals. The grandest was the Manchester Royal Infirmary, where I was first a student, and the 'lowliest' was a small cottage-type hospital in a Lancashire town. Even in those early days, I realized that the *rapport* and confidence between the patients and the medical staff in the local hospital was something I had never seen in the Manchester Royal Infirmary. But then, how could you compare the efficiency of one with the other? Well, after fifty years, I am still wondering which is the more important to the vast majority of patients, always excepting the need for technical efficiency by the surgeon in cases that can be cured. The remainder of the time was spent in doing locum work, i.e. deputizing for a general practitioner who was going on holiday, or working as an assistant in a busy practice.

In 1931 I married and bought a practice in Darwen, Lancashire, and that is where my story really begins.

I soon confirmed what I had already suspected, that the world of general practice was quite different from that of a medical student and house surgeon. There were tremendous differences in the types of cases, and also the reactions of the people seemed more important. Whereas in hospital one was used to seeing individual people with their own particular disease for which they were admitted, here, especially when visiting homes, one had to deal not only with the individual who was ill but also with the relatives. The difference was quite unnerving, and it was for this reason that I had a limited confidence in my ability to deal with people in these circumstances. I had not been trained to deal with human beings and families as such, but with individuals and their diseases. It might be more near the truth if I simply said 'diseases', for in those days the individual was scarcely considered. It took time to realize that there would have to be a reorientation of my ideas about disease.

Hospital training had brought me into contact with major diseases and illnesses, but these occurred only very infrequently in general practice. People were coming to see me with complaints which I did not understand because their symptoms did not fit into any of the diseases I had been taught. It was some time before I felt able to cope with these new problems. Gradually I classified them into four distinct groups:

1. The common infectious diseases, influenza, upper respiratory disease, allergy, teething and problems of constipation and pregnancy.
2. Major disease which could be diagnosed and treated.
3. Complaints which could not be diagnosed in terms of known disease.
4. Diseases which could be diagnosed but which had symptoms which did not improve sufficiently with the treatment of the disease originally diagnosed.

Apart from dealing with all these diseases and complaints as such, there was always the emotional problems of individuals and family to complicate them. It is important to realize that illness has this effect. It is part of human nature which has to be accepted, understood and properly evaluated.

As you will see later, increasing experience and knowledge enabled me to alter the original groupings. For the present, I would like to deal with them as they are. I think you will find it more interesting to see how and why the changes came about.

Within a period of six years the practice had grown so big that I found it impossible to give adequate time to each patient. It was quite clear that, once I stopped listening to, or examining, patients, the skills developed over my student years and the early years in practice would be blunted. As a result of this inevitable lowering of standards, I decided to give up the practice and go somewhere where people could afford to pay me for the time that must be spent, if a proper consideration of their symptoms was to be given. I also needed to learn much more about rheumatism and all these undiagnosable conditions which seemed vaguely linked with that indefinable disease.

During the time I was in this practice, I suggested and organized a rota-system between twelve of the doctors practising in the town, so that we were able to have our Sundays and half-days off without any anxiety regarding ourselves or our patients. It was already obvious that, without reasonable relaxation, our work became onerous and efficency impaired. This must have been the very first example of co-operation between a group of doctors in the country.

I left Darwen in 1937 and took a practice in Highgate, London. This practice was very small, so I was once again able to devote much more time to each patient. I also succeeded in obtaining an unpaid post as clinical assistant at the Charterhouse Rheumatism Clinic. I will be forever grateful to the late Dr Warren Crowe who founded the clinic, for the seventeen years I spent there researching amongst the countless numbers of rheumatic sufferers and from whom I learned so much, by listening and examining. I also worked at the Royal Homoeopathic Hospital as assistant to Mr W. E. Tucker, the orthopaedic surgeon, from whom I learned and was able to practise manipulative techniques, much of which was inspired by reading about osteopathy.

As a result of all this study, my practice grew and flourished, and in due time, following the war, I gave up most of my general-practice work and concentrated on the rheumatic diseases. I thus became a specialist in these diseases because of my interest and the challenge they presented.

This was not, of course, the orthodox way to become a specialist, although you might think it was logical. The orthodox method was to take an advanced degree in general medicine whilst doing junior hospital work and then to apply for a post in a hospital. Rheumatic departments were not very popular amongst potential specialists, and from the non-progress in the solution of their problems they do not seem to have attracted any outstanding contributors.

I hope my readers will have gathered from this chapter that I realized that medical education could and did teach very well all the diseases it knew about. Obviously, it could not do this about illness of which it was not aware. I was shocked to find how little knowledge was available to deal with the endless complaints which affected most people. I now realize that it was the urge to try to understand these problems which drove me to London in 1937. I do not regret the extra personal problems that the war caused me by forcing me to live in London, because I was able to pursue my studies.

I believed that I had brought some understanding into an area of illness which has never been properly charted, and in order to increase medical awareness of this mass of unsolved illness I published a number of papers:
'Social Aspect of Physical and Industrial Medicine' (*British Journal of Physical Medicine*, Volume VIII, no. 6, 1945)
'A Clinical Study of the Chronic Rheumatic Diseases and their Treatment by the Diptheroids' (*Journal of Rheumatism, January 1950*)
'The Value of Physiotherapy in the Treatment of Chronic Rheumatism' (*Medical Press*, Volume CCXXVIII, no. 5925, 1952)
'A New Approach to the Aetiology and Medical Treatment of Arthritis of the Hip' (*British Journal of Clinical Practice*, Volume XX, no. 12, 1966)
In 1975, believing I had achieved a sufficient knowledge and clarity, my book *Arthritis and Allied Conditions—A New and Successful Approach* was published. Although it was extremely well received by those members of the profession who read it (I append a number of reviews and opinions at

the end of this chapter), the Establishment chose to ignore it. The public, however, showed a remarkable interest in it, and with very limited non-medical publicity (i.e. London Broadcasting, *Vogue, Hampstead and Highgate Express* and *Darwen News*) requests for the book came from all over Britain, mainly through the public libraries. Because of this public interest, I have written this book for you all. The understanding of illness, which I hope you will get from it, should make communication between you and your doctor more intelligible and thus increase the chances of having your problems solved. Maybe it will stimulate more of the medical profession to ask why they were not made aware of my first book.

Reviews and Opinions of *Arthritis and Allied Conditions*

"Dr Fox's work and his excellent results are well known to me. It is remarkable the favourable response which occurs following the Fox method."
Maurice Lee, FRCS, Editorial Adviser, *What's New in Surgery*

"I want to congratulate you on a fine bit of original research and also on the results that you have achieved."
Rodney Maingot MS FRCS, Editor-in-Chief, *The British Journal of Clinical Practice.*

"The new approach will make a lasting contribution to this difficult subject. No practitioner whether general or specialist can fail to learn a great deal from this publication."
Albert Davis, MD FRCS, Consulting Surgeon, Prince of Wales Hospital, Tottenham and Bearsted Memorial Hospital.

"The author describes the results of his studies and methods of treatment over some forty years . . . written by a dedicated, confident physician who reveals his humanity in his writing."
E. M. Shipsey, the journal *Update Review*

"A new approach to the problem. All the signs, symptoms and histories have been brought together to give a coherent picture of the disease-process in the different forms of arthritis . . . treatment based on these findings gives uniformly good results."
Therapy

"I have used Dr Fox's method in nearly fifty cases. The results achieved are far better than I had hoped. Dr Fox has certainly justified the claims made in his book."
Dr John Clements, Dublin.

"Reading your book on arthritis was a real pleasure for me. I think you have a brilliant view upon the facts. I suffer from arthritis, and you have described exactly my whole life story."
Dr Luc Janssens, Hemiksem, Belgium.

2

The Problem

Consider that so many diseases have been cured or almost eradicated by antibiotics and vaccines, that people are far better fed, clothed and housed than ever before, that there is far more leisure and entertainment, and that we are living much longer, which must mean we are healthier. Furthermore, the medical services, with all their faults, are very freely and widely available. Does it not, therefore, seem paradoxical that we should require more and bigger hospitals, more and more equipment and a limitless budget?

What on earth is the matter with us? Have we developed a new set of diseases? Have we all become hypochondriacs, neurotics and drug-takers?

Well, of course, if you do not conform to the pattern of known disease, that is what can happen when you get into the endless belt of present-day medical practice. In my considered opinion, this state of affairs has come about because the art of medical diagnosis has been choked by 'medical science'. It stems from the false assumption that all forms of disease are recognizable and diagnosable and that the cause and cure of them is only a matter of scientific research. I believe this misconception has come about as a result of over-specialization in the study and teaching of disease.

There are at least twenty-five specialists dealing with the various illnesses that afflict the human race. You can have the services of a specialist in diseases of brain and spinal cord, lungs, heart, liver, kidney, glands, eyes, ear, nose and throat, skin, hair and nails, blood, bones, children, women's diseases, pregnancy, old age, arthritis, migraine, backache and psychiatry.

In all the various branches of medicine and surgery (apart from road accidents), the first contact with the medical services that a patient makes is with the general practitioner. In theory the doctor should be able to make an assessment of the complaint.

1. He knows what it is and how to deal with it, either by treatment or by referring the patient to the appropriate specialist.
2. He thinks he knows what it is, gives advice and treatment but keeps watch over the patient's progress. If the patient gets better, then the doctor might have been right, or recovery was spontaneous. In either case the result is satisfactory, so the patient and doctor are content.
3. The patient does not improve. Various remedies may have been tried with no success, or maybe the patient got better last time but on the next occasion does not respond to similar treatment.

Now the doctor begins to wonder what the patient is really suffering from. He has not been able to relieve the symptoms or to make a diagnosis.

Let us suppose the pain is in the abdomen. The doctor thought at first it was a stomach disorder or mild gallbladder disease, but you did not improve with diet or medicine. You are sent to a surgeon or physician who specializes in one or both of these suspected diseases. Examination, X-rays, blood-tests: all are negative. During this stage your symptoms may actually get better again, just as they did earlier on, and so no one is any longer concerned. Sooner or later the symptoms return: more investigations, more specialists, still no diagnosis. Every specialist you have seen confidently asserts you have not got the disease they specialize in.

Doubts are now creeping into the mind of your doctor, and even *you* begin to wonder about yourself! Are you imagining or exaggerating your symptoms? You have no language that can be intelligible to the doctor because you are just as confused as he or she. Some of you are even afraid to tell the doctor that you are no better. Are you now becoming slightly unstable or neurotic? Perhaps not un-expectedly, under the circumstances, you may be given a sedative or tranquillizer. This dulls your perception, makes the pain or discomfort more tolerable and may very well coincide with another period when your symptoms dis-appear—what we call a remission. How easy it is to ascribe it to the pill you are taking! Just as before, the medicine got the credit. But how tragic, for now you are docketed as psychosomatic or, even worse, as neurotic. Treatment for you in the future is endless pill-taking and perhaps psycho-therapy.

Of course, there are some patients who would not accept the situation. They might go to an acupuncturist, osteopath or any other of a dozen unorthodox practitioners. These practitioners will invariably restore confidence in yourself, a very valuable service, because they will give you an acceptable explanation of your condition. They are not charlatans, they believe what they tell you, and sometimes they are right, particularly the osteopath. In any case, you are by now due for a further remission of your symptoms, and, just as with the doctor, whatever treatment you are receiving at the time is given the credit for the cure. I will be discussing this aspect in a later chapter.

The failure of the profession to diagnose your case is simply due to the fact that every specialist you have seen says, "No, you have not got a disease." But where is the doctor who gives credence to your complaints, who asks, "Has this patient got symptoms we do not understand, and is there an underlying condition we do not know about?" I am afraid there are very few doctors who question the adequacy of their knowledge or seek for an explanation of symptoms which do not fit into a recognizable disease.

Let us see if we can learn anything from the history of medicine. The art of clinical medicine was laid down centuries ago. It was the result of observations by intelligent and enquiring minds of barber surgeons, herbalists and other practitioners who later developed into doctors. They tried to correlate the patients' complaints (symptoms) with the visible manifestations of the disease, such as a rash, swelling or loss of movement (signs) and what they found on examination of the body. To this was added the history of any previous complaints, and thus was formed the case-history of the patient. All known diseases were the result of this meticulous documentation, and one can only wonder at the remarkable achievements of men whose knowledge of anatomy and physiology (how the body functions) was comparatively rudimentary.

Having arrived at a diagnosis, they tried to treat the patient with a limited number of drugs, the actions of which were not well understood. Bearing in mind that they did not understand the disease, it could not be surprising that there was a great deal of speculation and disagreement about its cause and the methods of treatment. In the main, treatment resolved itself into trying to reverse symptoms, such as by a purge if there was constipation, or with something to stop the motions if there was diarrhoea. There were other methods, such as blood-letting, leeches, hot and cold compresses, depending on what the doctors thought might help the victim. We now know that treatment was mostly ineffectual, if not sometimes positively harmful, and the death or recovery of the patient was really due to the failure or success of the patient's own natural resistance.

You can now see that, where a disease was not really understood, treatment was based on the counteraction or suppression of symptoms. It was not very scientific, but it was all they could do in those days.

Many of you may have read or seen Bernard Shaw's play *The Doctor's Dilemma*. Cleverly and wittily, it posed the problems of the cause and treatment of disease at the expense of the doctors. Nevertheless, Shaw failed to appreciate their difficulties or to recognize the remarkable progress which had been made in the art of diagnosis.

The explanation of how and why these diseases arose and how to treat them developed from speculation to scientific discoveries in physiology (the study of body functions), bacteriology (the study of germs) and pathology (the effect of the disease on body tissues). Investigative techniques, such as blood- and electrical tests and X-rays, have multiplied the ways in which diseases can be more clearly analysed in order to establish or disprove an exact diagnosis. As a result of this scientific research, the actual causes of many diseases were discovered. They were mostly germs of various types, and the prevention or cure of the disease was effected by public health measures, vaccines and antibiotics. Examples about which we all know are typhoid, pneumonia, tuberculosis, venereal disease and poliomyelitis. There are other diseases involving various glands in the body which became amenable to precise hormone or drug treatment, such as thyroid and pituitary diseases. These successes were due to the fact that the scientific tests done in the laboratory corresponded with the original clinical picture of the disease. The scientists had served the clinicians well precisely because they had been presented with a coherent clinical story.

Following these achievements, it then seemed reasonable to believe that further scientific investigations would solve all our remaining problems. This, I suggest, is where we have gone wrong.

Up till now, all the scientific investigations were directed towards finding the cause of a disease about which all the details were known and fully comprehended. For example pneumonia, typhoid and many other infectious diseases were so well tabulated in their case-histories that there was substantially no doubt about the diagnosis or the clinical story. Scientists isolated the germ, and they found an antibiotic to kill it. When we come to such diseases as rheumatism and arthritis, the problem is quite different. Clinicians do not understand how the disease begins, how or why it varies in severity and what actually causes it. They have described different forms of these diseases, such as rheumatoid arthritis, osteo-arthritis and spondylitis and do not know if they have a common origin or not. We have masses of facts and no understanding. Therefore, the scientists who are investigating this problem have no clear clinical indication as to where they should direct their energies and indeed what they should be looking for.

This statement is so fundamental to the study of disease that some examples of what I mean are worth describing now.

Almost every patient with arthritis has some blood-tests done as a routine. Two examples are the sedimentation-rate and the rheumatoid factor; neither of them is particularly reliable, and they contribute nothing to the understanding of the disease. X-rays are done routinely and often repeated at regular intervals; again, they can tell you nothing more than an intelligent clinical examination will reveal. Short-wave and ultrasonic equipment for the treatment of joints is just an expensive way of directing heat, which, apart from the psychological and comforting effects, have very little curative value. All these 'scientific' agencies are the stock in trade of the rheumatologists which help to perpetuate the myth that they know much more than general practitioners, who are just as capable of prescribing the same anti-rheumatic drugs as they use. These drugs are all produced by scientists who are trying to produce a cure for diseases which they do not understand, and that is why there is this endless flow of them, none of which has the slightest hope of real success.

A further example of this scientific waste is in the recent report by the media of a scientist who claims that tissue-typing will help to determine which patients are likely to get rheumatoid arthritis and that this, in some mysterious way, is going to help solve the problem! If he really understood the early symptoms of this disease, he would not need tissue-typing to know who was going to get it—he would recognize it long before the rheumatologist. What might be more useful is to tissue-type people who do not develop the disease and try to find out why they are not susceptible. In any event, in order to make any real sense of the theory, you have to postulate a starting-factor, and this scientist thinks it might be a virus. Can you see that this work, although scientifically based, lacks direction?

What I have said about arthritis, which we recognize only when it is advanced, applies to many other complaints that have been labelled with a name which means and signifies no knowledge beyond the literal translation of the word. For example, 'coxalgia' means pain related to an area of bone at the lower end of the spine called the coccyx; 'brachial neuralgia' means a pain relating to a section of the nervous system going to the arm. These terms and many others, such as 'fibrositis', 'tennis elbow', 'migraine' and 'sprains', have been in common medical usage for so long that they have been accorded, albeit unintentionally, the status of a diagnosis, because patients accept these names of their complaints as implying that the doctors understand their disease, which, of course, the GPs will be the first to admit that they do not. There are many other complaints, such as 'indeterminate pains' in the stomach or chest, for which doctors cannot even think of a name, never mind a diagnosis, simply because they cannot relate them to known diseases.

Herein lies the very real danger of the patients being labelled psychosomatic, neurotic or even psychological. They are the ones who are given tranquillizers or similar drugs which dull their mental ability and may even alter their personality. In view of all the knowledge and resources we have, I submit that this form of 'treatment' is worse and more harmful than anything used in the bygone days which inspired *The Doctor's Dilemma*.

In the name of progress we have built up a massive organization of investigative techniques. Their original intention was to help elucidate the problems of known diseases and to confirm the disease in its earlier stages when all the clinical details had not yet developed. The value of these activities can be seen in preventative medicine, as in suspected typhoid and the ability to treat serious diseases such as cancer and diabetes at a much earlier stage. Unfortunately, they are used far too frequently for the investigation not of a known or suspected disease based on clinical knowledge but of an isolated symptom or complaint which vaguely resembles a known disease, the types of cases to which I have just referred. This is a prostitution of clinical medicine because the investigations can tell you only that it is, or is not, the disease you suspect but cannot tell you anything about the complaint if the results are negative. In my experience, which is not inconsiderable, only a small fraction of the investigation done in hospitals produces positive results. Here is the real nub of the tragedy—no one can find a physical explanation for your complaint. Have they not used every possible modern invention to solve your case? Is it any wonder that you are viewed with suspicion by all and sundry?

With a better clinical understanding of these cases, a significant part of this great waste of talent, time and materials could be eliminated, and scientific medicine could resume its proper function, to elucidate the causes of diseases we understand clinically and not to give negative information on diseases or symptoms we do not understand.

The profession has come to rely on X-rays, blood-tests, etc, to solve these problems. By adopting this method of 'progress', they fail to develop their clinical acumen beyond the stage of their student days. In this way they have built a mental wall against increasing the clinical understanding of disease. Because they can see no further than this wall, they rely on scientific investigations to probe its foundations, to analyse the atmosphere around it and maybe to drill a small hole here and there which gives insufficient vision of what is beyond. How much more logical and simpler to build another step or two on the ladder of clinical facts, which would then enable us to see over this wall and so have a clearer vision of what is there! It is because they think they have all the clinical facts that this progress is not made.

If it should be doubted that this latter statement does not represent a true assessment of the present clinical attitude of the specialist, let me refer you to the efforts being directed to achieve computer diagnosis in other countries as well as our own.

The very idea that a machine can produce a diagnosis more efficiently than a doctor suggests that there may not be too much confidence in the diagnostic ability of the profession as a whole. I know that this statement can be argued against on the grounds of time-saving, but it does not invalidate the point I am making. Everybody associated with computers knows that the machine can give you answers only on the facts with which you feed it. It cannot deduce that there are facts missing which would complete the picture; it can merely give you an incomplete one. In other words, it cannot tell you any more than you already know. That is why the computer recently developed at Glasgow University failed to improve on already accepted knowledge and diagnosis. I believe the cost for each case investigated was about £1,000—it may have been time-saving, but it was certainly very expensive. I am quite sure that the doctors concerned know very well that the success of the computer must depend on giving the full data, for otherwise they would not have used it. Does this not confirm what I have already said? They think they know all there is to know about the clinical facts of the disease and that science, the computer, will provide the answers.

So I repeat: they do not know all the facts and can collect them only by diligent clinical investigation. That is what my book was based on.

When medical successes were achieved, I rejoiced with everyone else, but always in my mind was the conscious-ness of our failure to understand and treat the vast mass of sufferers who filled the waiting-rooms in general practice and the hospitals. This failure must continue until such time as we can produce doctors who have both the clinical interest and the time to devote to the study of these patients. The education and training of doctors have been devised by specialists in almost every branch of medical learning, and none can deny their knowledge and ability. However, the specialists do not come in contact with, nor are they particularly interested in, any cases outside their discipline. The newly qualified doctors are a product of this system and, therefore, perpetuate these attitudes. Specific-ally, they fail to consider and interpret symptoms which do not fit into the diseases they know.

We must, therefore, return to the Art of Medicine, listen to the patients, collect and collate all their case-histories and, like the great clinicians of the past, present a coherent clinical picture. Only then can the scientist make a positive contribution.

The art and science of medicine have been built on the study of people who are ill. They, unlike animals (of which we use far too many), can speak—so why do we not listen to them more? This is precisely what I have always done. My laboratory has been the consulting-room—my tools have been an enquiring mind and sensitive fingers, trained in the skills taught to me as a student. Empathy, humility and logic gave me the ability to listen and then relate the patients' stories with the clinical findings. Thus I have built up a coherent clinical picture which explains so many of those symptoms which cannot be integrated into present-day recognizable disease-patterns.

Because medical education is based on all the known specialities, there is no specialist who can identify with my new findings. Because general practitioners are trained by those same specialists, they lack the ability to comprehend that which they have never been taught. Only the handful of specialists and GPs who have had experience of my work know that what I am saying is true. There are many patients who can also bear witness to my claims, and I have little doubt that many of my readers will find themselves slotting into some of the categories described.

3

The New Clinical Picture:
Problem of Diagnosis

With increasing study and experience I was able to reclassify all patients in Groups 3 and 4.

Group A: Patients of all ages, but more frequent as they grew older, complaining of pains in various parts of the body which, depending on the site of the pain, were called sprains, stiff neck, pleurodymia, lumbago, sciatica, coxalgia, brachial neuralgia, tennis elbow, fibrositis or, if a joint was obviously affected, arthritis. Treatment varied according to the severity or persistence of the symptoms, from aspirin to a large variety of rheumatic drugs, liniments, rest, heat, massage, exercises, etc. None of them was in any sense curative, and they were merely palliatives (sometimes ill-advised) until natural recovery took place.

Group B: These patients had pains in the head—headache or migraine; pains over the heart which might give rise to suspicion of angina; pains in other parts of the chest suggesting pleurisy or other chest diseases; pains over the abdominal area vaguely resembling liver or gall-bladder discomfort, perhaps chronic appendix or kidney disease.

Group C: These were the relatively small number of patients who had a diagnosable disease but where improvement was not as good as it should be with the treatment given. They had the diagnosed disease and in addition some factor in common with Group B.

At that time it was impossible for me to see these groups so clearly, and I could not really relate them to the growing number of arthritics which developed as the years went by. What was important at that time was the realization that I did not understand all this conglomeration of complaints simply because they were not taught in the medical schools or hospitals—nobody had studied or analysed them. I resolved to try to get some order out of this chaos. It has taken nearly forty years. I know many of you will recognize your own symptoms in this story, and maybe it will help arouse more interest in what is immediately possible to relieve a considerable amount of unnecessary suffering, by being able to make a correct diagnosis.

I have never believed that people go to doctors because they have nothing better to do. They go because they feel ill or have a pain, and who is wise enough to measure this? Of course, there are some people—I believe, relatively few—who have unresolved psychological problems and use the pain or discomfort as a peg on which to place the responsibility. This is quite different from the psychological problems which may be caused by the doctor not understanding the reason for the pain, discomfort and ill-health of the genuine sufferer.

Let us start with a picture which many women, in particular in the twenty-to-forty age-group, will recognize. You are feeling quite well and coping with all the problems of housekeeping, looking after the children and perhaps doing a job. You get up one morning full of aches, tired and depressed. Like most normal people, you try to ignore it and get on with your work. Perhaps you try an aspirin or some other advertised drug and feel better. In a day or two it is all over, and you are back to normal and forget all about it. As time goes by, you get further attacks; the intervals can vary from weeks to months, or even years. The longer the intervals, the less likely you are to remember them, which is natural and sensible, and the less likely they are to have inflicted any permanent damage on your body.

Now we come to the people who are not so fortunate. The attack lasts for more than a day or two and does not respond to the home or advertised remedies. The tiredness and aching persist, the chores become more difficult to cope with, and the depression starts to take hold. You have no real pains or any other visible signs which would account for your condition. The children do not understand, and your husband might or might not be sympathetic. You go to the doctor, and in no time at all he has prescribed a tonic or some other medicine. Sometimes you feel better, and sometimes you do not. When you do, both you and your doctor are pleased, until the next bout occurs and the prescription does not work. When you do not improve, in spite of the various medicines, it then becomes 'tension' or 'neurosis', and the tranquillizers make their *début*. These dull your perceptions, and you may feel less depressed and try to carry on, but your condition persists.

What in fact has happened is that none of the treatment has had any curative effect, and the disease has gone through its natural behaviour of getting worse and then better, what the doctors call 'relapses' and 'remissions'—when they recognize them. As time goes by, the periods of relapses (feeling worse) become longer, and the periods of remission (feeling better) become shorter.

In due course the general aching and feeling below par become obscured in the mind because: (a) you get used to a lower standard of health facilitated by pain-relieving drugs or tranquillizers, or both (frequently); (b) there is a development of more definite pains located in one or more areas, say in the hand or knee; it could, of course, develop anywhere. Later these painful episodes are associated with some limitation of movement and also with stiffness, particularly after resting for longish periods. If they have not already occurred, cramp in the hands or feet becomes another problem, particularly in the middle of the night. The next stage is a precisely located pain, more marked limitation of movement and swelling of a joint where this is visible, i.e. hands or feet. At this point it does not require a genius to diagnose arthritis, and by this time there may be X-ray evidence of early arthritis.

Many of you in the age-group referred to remember having pains in the knees or thighs when at school, or recurrent backache before the onset of the menstrual period? You may have children who are having the same problems, all rather transient and forgettable but a sure indication of the continuity of the rheumatic story. I must stress that arthritis is not inevitable, as many people develop an immunity to the disease. I am concerned only about the people whose episodes of illness and pain become more persistent, and the intervals of good health become shorter. Unless you are in this category, there is no need to be worried. Nature, given half a chance, is on your side, and even in the deteriorating cases it will co-operate with the right understanding and treatment.

How many of you have been sent to hospital because of pain in the back, the hands or the feet, had blood-tests and X-rays and been told there is no arthritis? So if you have no arthritis, what are you fussing about? Even so, you are given all kinds of rheumatic drugs which, whilst giving relief to some, do nothing to make you better. How many of you have children who complain of headache, pain in an arm or leg, or even tummyache, which seem bad enough to go to the doctor? Of course you do not bother with a transient pain which you and the child soon forget about. It is the pain that persists or the feeling of illness, which most parents instinctively know about their children, which makes you consult the doctor. The same story is again repeated. Try some medicine—heaven knows what. If the child gets better, that is OK for the time being. If not, off you are sent to hospital: the same routine of examination, investigation and no diagnosis.

What I have been trying to explain to the medical profession in my book is that arthritis, recognizable by X-ray, takes a long time to develop and is a result of the disease which has been attacking the body through all the years of aching, tiredness and depression. Where the condition develops rapidly (that is, in a year or two), it generally becomes what we call rheumatoid arthritis—the most severe of them all. Where the development is much slower, and it can be more than twenty years, it tends to fall into the category of osteo-arthritis. In between, you get cases which are referred to as mixed rheumatoid and osteo-arthritis. We also know that countless cases which are X-rayed for chest or stomach diseases in adults show osteo-arthritis of the spine which has given no *remembered* symptoms of pain in the back previously. That arthritis has taken many years to develop. If these patients are closely questioned, they almost always recall pains or aching in the back or vague chest or stomach pains in the distant past. Where these X-rays prove negative for disease of the lungs and abdomen, the answer to their problem may very well be in arthritis of the spine. These types are the ones we shall be discussing in Group B.

Now let us return to the earlier symptoms which have plagued you for years. What do they mean? Quite simply they are symptoms of a general infection like influenza in a mild form. During the long years of my investigations, I arranged for many patients to take their temperatures during these achy and depressed days. A high percentage of them showed a rise in temperature of ½–1°F during the day, which often, but not always, fell to normal or below in the morning after a night in bed. Some of you will also recall mild sweating of the hands or feet during these periods, and a considerable number will recall that the onset of their first attack was preceded by influenza or sore throat, possibly two or three weeks before.

All these facts which I have described, aching, tiredness, depression, very slightly raised temperature and mild sweating, add up to an undoubted medical picture of a low-grade influenza-like infection, as distinct from acute infections such as the various fevers, pneumonias or obvious cases of influenza. This kind of low-grade infection has never been recognized or described in medical textbooks. It should not, therefore, be in the least surprising that it is not realized that these symptoms represent the early stages of a rheumatic disease. Furthermore, when the doctors are unaware of the rise in temperature—the only piece of objective evidence in favour of some physical illness, they are left with tiredness, depression and achiness to consider. Well, what else would you expect from a married woman with two or three children, a home to look after, problems of making ends meet, perhaps doing an extra job herself, and a husband whose personal and sexual demands may be more than she can cope with? The diagnosis must be tension or neurosis. Another diagnostic failure—another case for tranquillizers and the psychiatric junk-heap. In a later chapter I will give you examples which have occurred in my own practice.

At this point I would like to make some observation about colds. As you all know, many millions of pounds have been spent on research into the cause of colds, or, as it is called by the establishment, coryza. Blind the public with a Latin word and call it a diagnosis! They have found a considerable number of different viruses over the years as the cause, and they have isolated a substance, Inteferon, which will 'cure' the cold—at a cost of about £1,000 per person.

Now let me put the cold or coryza problem in simple terms which any lay person can understand. Germs and viruses are everywhere. They are looking for breeding-grounds. The human body happens to be a happy hunting-ground for some of them. They enter the nasal passages and immediately start to invade the lining or mucous membrane. If they succeed, they can penetrate the defences and get into the body cells, which they prefer. These cells may be nerve, liver, kidney, lung or connective tissues. It is these people who become ill with various diseases, some of which we can recognize as influenza, hepatitis, nephritis, sleeping-sickness and, I believe but cannot prove, multiple sclerosis. If, however, the body reacts against the virus, then you get a streaming cold, you feel rotten for a day or two, and then all is well. In other words, you have won the fight against the invader and developed an immunity to that virus.

If you look at it in this way, you will see one of the facets of the survival of the fittest, the development of resistance to disease, and this should be welcomed by the profession and not looked upon as a disease. By all means investigate any phenomenon. But do it for the right reason, and the answer will be all the more readily ascertained.

Another interesting fact I discovered by listening to my patients was that many people suffering from rheumatoid arthritis would remember that they used to have colds in their earlier life, but since the rheumatoid arthritis started, they have been free from them.

This was another important clinical fact suggesting that, if the disease has a viral origin, of which I am now quite sure, then it entered the body when the normal defence failed; there was no resistance, therefore no cold. Once the virus was settled in the cells of its choice, then the severity of the disease would depend on subsequent development of resistance (antibodies) in the patient. Some of the clinical evidence I had for this interpretation was that many of the arthritic patients had periods of great lassitude, aching and a small rise in temperature so reminiscent of influenza, associated with a further extension of the disease in the body, with some of the earliest-affected places getting worse.

What I have been describing in this chapter is a disease-process which can start in childhood or at any later stage. It can be mild and transient, severe and persistent, or any gradation between these two extremes. In the worst cases you get rheumatoid arthritis of varying severity which develops into a recognizable condition within one or two years. In the more slowly developing cases, you get the osteo-arthritic group which can take from around ten to twenty years to become recognizable. There are also those who may get better before any arthritis has time to develop. It is as though you have a film-sequence which can be made unrecognizable, except to those who know it, by running the film too quickly or too slowly, by over-exposure or under-exposure, by bad focusing or by stopping it altogether at any particular moment. You have to remember that all diseases vary in this way. Think of the children with whooping-cough, measles and chickenpox. Some have them so mildly you hardly recognize them, whilst others are so ill it is almost unbelievable. Before antibiotics, pneumonia presented the same variations, and a large number ended in death. Cancer shows the same variations—some develop quickly and some very slowly.

In following chapters evidence will be given which will, I hope, help you to understand and to believe what I know to be true, i.e. that all those complaints listed in Groups A and B are basically the same disease which in very many cases can be successfully treated. I repeat once again that the problem can be finally solved only when the medical pundits grasp the message, when the real scientific investigations are given the right direction.

4

The Rheumatic Patch

As a doctor, I found it impossible to deny all this clinical evidence of an infectious process, and so I pursued my investigations. Being now convinced that pain and some restriction of movement, the second stage of the disease-process, precede any swelling or arthritic changes in the joints, I examined in detail the areas of pain near the joints.

The most important discovery I made was the existence of small areas of pain and swelling underneath the skin in the connective tissue. This connective tissue is like an 'internal skin' which is in close contact with the muscles, tendons and joints and is loosely connected to the inside of the skin. Its functions have not been exactly determined, but I think that it probably contributes in a greater degree than is generally thought to the stabilization and move-ment of the muscles and joints. It is this tissue which becomes inflamed during the early attack. If you are lucky, the inflammation settles down and leaves no obvious damage, and so you recover. Often the patch remains dormant and becomes reactivated by a later attack. In other cases these small areas of inflammation persist and give rise to intermittent pain or aching which may later affect the nearby joints. I have confirmed the existence of these areas by taking samples of connective tissue from five different cases: two cases of rheumatoid arthritis, one of osteo-arthritis and two in which there was no X-ray evidence of arthritis but all other symptoms existed.

I want at this moment to try to convey to you that this investigation represented a crisis-point of my work. I had taken three different diseases as described in medical text-books, represented in five different people who were under my care at that particular time.

I explained to the pathologist, a highly reputable doctor, what I wanted to do and hoped to prove. I said that if all my clinical research and the deductions I had made from it were correct, then all these cases should show the same evidence of disease of the connective tissue under the microscope. He agreed that if it turned out as I predicted, it would constitute good evidence. I removed the tiny pieces of tissue under local anaesthetic from each patient and labelled them only with the initials of the patient. The pathologist did not know who they were or what their diseases were. The five reports were identical; the disease-process was the same in all the cases. If they had been really different, I might have lapsed into total silence. As it is, I now confidently describe these areas.

I call them 'rheumatic patches', and they are present in all cases of proven arthritis and in those earlier cases where the X-rays are negative. These patches are the ones which cause pain when pressed on by the hand of the examining doctor. Up till now these pains were thought to be due to tender-ness in the muscles (myalgia) or strangulated bits of fat (fat-herniation) or inflammation in or around the joints themselves (capulitis). The identification of these patches offers a simple and logical explanation for the pain, stiffness and limitation of movement in any part of the body. A considerable number of patients have been greatly improved by treating these patches, and the immediate results are predictable in *every* case. The long-term results depend on other factors which are all dealt with in the book. What I wish to stress now is that these patches, when related to the patients' symptoms, explain the clinical picture in all the rheumatic diseases.

You will understand much better what I am saying if you will study this diagram, which shows the different tissues to which I refer.

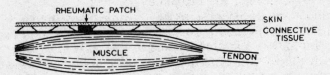

Between the skin and the connective tissue are some wavy lines which represent the strands of a loose connection between them. This allows freedom of movement of the skin and connective tissue in whichever direction they need to move, and I believe the strands are the medium through which the necessary information is passed. The muscle has its own covering or sheath which is similar to the connective tissue and in very close association with it. The sheath extends to and becomes part of the tendon of the muscle. The tendon is the part of the muscle which does the pulling when the muscle contracts—say, to raise the arm. All these tissues are alive and aware of each other, and they work in total harmony so that you are never conscious of them.

Now see what happens when a rheumatic patch arrives. It settles in the connective tissue in one area. The inflammation causes a reaction by the local tissues. Swelling and stickiness occur, and the affected part of the connective tissue gets stuck to the skin above it and possibly to the sheath of the muscle under it. It is an area which has become over-sensitive and painful. When you try to move the arm, it will move only until the affected area is called upon to do its part. It is at this point that pain and discomfort stop any further movement.

Here is an example. In this outline, the patient can raise the arm no further than you can see. What stops her is a pain, tightness or discomfort at Point A. If you examine this area, you will find that the skin is stuck to the underlying connecting tissue. It is tender to touch or pressure. If this area is injected with a local anaesthetic, the pain is abolished, and then it is possible to raise the arm much higher.

This proves three things: (1) there is an area of pain which I describe as a 'rheumatic patch'; (2) by abolishing the pain, the arm can be freed of the restricted movement; (3) there cannot possibly be anything wrong with the shoulder joint, otherwise you would not get increased painless movement.

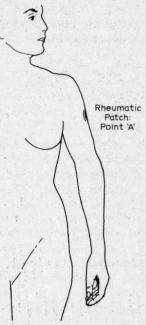

Rheumatic Patch: Point 'A'

The next question to be answered is, how do these patches first begin? Try to imagine the sandy beach by the sea. The sand represents the connective tissue. It covers and ramifies into the pebbles and earth under it. These represent the muscles, tendons and joints in the body. The air over the beach will represent the skin, which in this case you can see through. The sea represents the air we breathe, and in it is an oil-slick which represents the germs. The tide comes in, envelopes the sand and follows it down to its ramifications, and some of the oil gets through with the water. If you are lucky, it gets washed out again when the tide recedes. You have beaten the germs, and no harm is done. If, however, some of the oil sticks, then you get polluted areas, or in my terms rheumatic patches. You may have only one, so that you hardly noticed it getting in, or you can have several—the more you have, the worse the pollution or disease. The five cases I investigated were very heavily polluted and would need a great deal of cleansing (treatment). The very early and mild cases will have perhaps only one or two spots to start with. This may be sufficient to alert the defences against any subsequent attacks and to give the body time to dispose of the first spots. There may be no more pollution for some considerable time. Nobody has bothered to clean up the first mess, and now a second one arrives, adding a little more pollution. You can see how it will mount up after a time. In due course, it will clog up the works in various parts—that is, when the arthritis develops into its recognizable form.

If you have followed this explanation, you can begin to understand how an isolated pain in an arm or a leg, or indeed anywhere in the body, can be caused in exactly the same way as the widespread disease of rheumatoid or osteo-arthritis. I think it worthwhile repeating at this point that the first attack of rheumatism can start at any age. Possibly the earliest that could be clinically recognized is 'growing pains' in the knees or legs at ages four to five years. The patch which caused the pain developed possibly after one of the common fevers such as measles, chickenpox or a sore throat. Certainly the child had been 'off colour' for a day or two. As so often happens, it settles after a few days and is soon forgotten. You must not look upon these patches as being static (by which I mean unchanging— nothing to do with electricity). They are part of living tissue and are likely to have a virus in them. The virus and the inflammation caused by it may gradually be subdued and give rise to some localized scar-tissue, or the patches will get bigger and spread as the disease gets worse. They not only spread along the connective tissue close to the skin, they also appear to develop threads which spread inwards and become enmeshed with tendons and the sheaths covering the muscles, but also on to the capsule and ligaments near the joints. This is how arthritis first begins and spreads, so that the joints are the last part of the body to be invaded. Just finding the rheumatic patches does not necessarily mean that you can cure the symptoms. What it does mean is that you can explain why the symptoms have arisen and why the pain is where it is.

To cure the condition you must find the cause of the patches. On every possible occasion I want to repeat what I believe, i.e. that a virus causes the patches which are certainly areas of inflammation. If scientific research, which would include the use of an electron microscope, was concentrated on these patches in all their different stages of development, I am confident we should solve the whole problem of arthritis. In the meantime, your own body is not exactly asleep—all the force it is capable of is exerted to overcome the disease, and that is why in so many cases the patient improves in due time. I know from experience that many patients can be helped with treatment based on a realization of the true behaviour of the disease. Because it needs medical knowledge and expertise, I cannot offer you any simple advice. When members of the profession have studied my book, they will be in a position to provide the treatment I have been using.

It is important to realize that the first sign of any localized rheumatic patch is pain of varying intensity and duration. It is nearly always of sudden onset and without apparent cause. Sometimes the patient will recall, if asked, that it might have been preceded by a vague discomfort or ache which he hardly noticed, or he may have felt unwell some-time before. This is the time when the doctor, if only he was aware of it, would find the first rheumatic patch. You, the patient, if not in too much pain and if you are sufficiently inquisitive, can locate the spot yourself. It is very sensitive, but by compressing it between your thumb and fingers you can get a temporary relief of the pain and confirmation that my description is accurate.

Rheumatic cases declare themselves quite frequently by recurring sprains in different parts of the arms or legs or back. When these people do not improve, they move from doctor to hospital, to specialist and physiotherapist. After exhausting the medical services, they often move to osteo-paths, acupuncturists or other unorthodox practitioners. Somewhere along the line the condition suddenly improves because of the body's natural recuperative powers. What-ever treatment is being used at that time gets the credit for the 'cure'. If the patient is still in orthodox hands, you hear no more about it because a cure is what people expect and accept from the medical profession. If the improvement occurs whilst under treatment by an unorthodox practitioner, such as an osteopath or acupuncturist, and should the patient be in the public eye—well, that is news. The media gobble it up, and another unorthodox celebrity is born, only to sink into relative obscurity when the failures begin to tot up.

Now let me give you some examples which many of you will recognize. You are doing a simple job which you have done hundreds of times before, lifting a pan off the stove or using a screwdriver. Suddenly, your wrist gets painful, and you think "Ah! I have sprained it." You have to stop what you are doing, rest the wrist, perhaps bandage it, and in a day or two it is better, and you forget about it. If it is very painful and does not settle fairly quickly, you go to the doctor. He confirms it is a sprain, gives you some liniment or whatever, and in due course you get better. The real diagnosis and the question of rheumatism have never arisen.

The same confusion can arise when an ankle is affected. In this case, you think you have tripped over a stair or pavement, when in fact your foot has given way because of a sudden rheumatic attack. The same story as the wrist is repeated. Of course, you can trip over a stair or a pavement and do yourself an injury when you have no rheumatism. In these cases, you can get up and start walking normally if there is no severe injury, otherwise there is pain, bruising and swelling to confirm the real injury. None of these do you find if rheumatism is the cause. You may, of course, trip because of rheumatism and cause injury to the ankle area with bruising and swelling. Now you suffer the effect of two conditions—the rheumatic condition and the injury. These are the cases which take much longer than expected to get better because the injury aggravates the rheumatism, and the rheumatism delays the normal recovery process. The recovery is even further delayed when it is not realized that there is a rheumatic area present, because the next stage in the treatment for this injury is heat, massage and exercises. The heat can do little harm, but the massage and exercises will only aggravate the inflamed rheumatic patch. These kinds of problems, whether affecting the wrist, elbow, ankle or knee, are common.

Then there is the ever-recurring 'tennis elbow'. Why should any athlete who is repeating the same movement of the arm, at a time when he is trained to an absolute peak, suddenly develop a sprain or pulled muscle or tendon. 'Tennis elbow' is just a name to describe a disability of the elbow and does not mean that the cause of it is understood. But a rheumatic area would soon explain the whole problem, and correct diagnosis and treatment would provide an early, if only temporary, solution of the symptoms.

I mention these types of case now because I am not normally consulted at this stage—the situation is much worse when I see the patient. By delving back into the histories of arthritic cases, these episodes have been recalled, but they have never before been associated with their present condition.

All other types of case will be demonstrated in case-reports in later chapters.

5

Other Factors which Affect Rheumatic Areas

I hope you will now understand my thesis that rheumatism is an inflammation of certain body-tissues (mainly connective tissue) which is caused in part by a virus. It is true that so far none has ever been isolated, but I have given you reasons why I believe success can be achieved.

In the treatment of every case there are a number of other factors which have to be taken into consideration. This diagram contains them all.

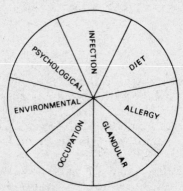

There may be only one or two applicable to any particular

case, but it is important that they be treated. You will see why as I deal with them. Remember that I consider infection by virus to be present in every case, so I will deal with that in the next chapter when I discuss specific treatment for all rheumatic diseases.

DIET. There are two aspects of diet which can be discussed. The first is the actual amounts of food we eat and the calories they represent. The importance of this form of diet in arthritis has been overstressed, although it could be advantageous to a patient to diet if grossly overweight. It will, however, do nothing to help combat the disease. Many patients with arthritis put on weight because of the enforced idleness, which in turns causes boredom, a very potent cause of over-eating, especially if they do not smoke! Most people's diet is probably adequate in vitamins, but because of the infective and debilitating nature of the disease, plus the adverse effects of so much drug-taking, the more ill patients can be helped by a short and intensive course of vitamins—mainly B and C given by injection into a vein. A vitamin C supplement of 500 mg daily is certainly worth taking during the active stage of the disease.

   The second aspect of diet has to be understood in terms of items of food which disagree with the patient in the obvious ways, when they say "I don't like" this or that, or when they cause a feeling of nausea, stomach-upset or diarrhoea. There are less obvious ways, which should prove not too difficult for you or the doctor to detect, such as rashes, urticaria in a mild or severe form and even very obscure examples of intolerance to milk, cheese and chocolate which have been found in some cases of headaches, migraine, etc. All these examples are due to what we call allergy, and they will be considered in that respect.

ALLERGY. This is a condition an obvious example of which must be known to almost every person in the land. I refer to hay fever. It is caused by pollen from plants, trees and flowers carried in the air, which causes severe irritation of the mucous membranes in the eyes, nose and throat of the sufferer. Another example is dermatitis of the hands, which may be caused by a detergent or other irritating substances where the skin has cracked, scratched or cut. Unlike hay fever, the protective layer of skin has to be pierced before the irritant can do any harm.

A third type of allergy is a rash suddenly affecting the skin after eating some food which acts as a poison. The rash is called urticaria and can occur after eating strawberries, mushrooms and many other foods which cannot always be identified. The common characteristic in all these types is an outpouring of fluid—in hay fever the watering of the eyes and nose, in dermatitis the weeping of the skin, and in urticaria the wheals of the rash which contain fluid.

A great number of rheumatic sufferers provide evidence of one or other form of these allergies, and I believe the swelling around the joints has an element of allergy in it. These examples of allergy are the more obvious and therefore the more easily recognizable ones. The more obscure cases are those to which I referred earlier. The question of allergy must be considered in every case of rheumatic disease, because in the present state of our knowledge it is impossible to deny the importance of the role of the allergic state, in either making the body tissues more susceptible to a virus attack or in enhancing the damage that a virus or any other inflammatory agent may initiate. Because allergy is a specialist subject of Dr Freed's, he has instigated a research project into the behaviour of the cells in the rheumatic patches taken from my own cases. Perhaps by the time this book reaches you, we may have more to tell you.

Meanwhile, because almost every rheumatic sufferer will provide some evidence of allergy when carefully questioned and examined, I consider it mandatory to deal with it from the very onset. When it is possible to do this quickly and easily in the obvious cases, there is no real problem. Because of the difficulty with the more obscure cases, it is best to use a mild anti-histamine in all cases. It undoubtedly reduces discomfort and irritation at night, of which so many patients complain. It allows them to rest and sleep much better without taking sleeping-tablets or tranquillizers. The drug is quite harmless. In some patients it may give rise to a temporary dryness in the mouth, a slight difficulty in focusing or a little drowsiness. For this reason I recommend that the tablet or capsule be taken only in the evening, an hour or two before bedtime, so that these side-effects will have passed off by mid-morning. The dose I use is Phenergan 10 mgs or capsules Benadryl 25 mgs—the latter having a slower and more sustained action which I prefer. These drugs have been taken by my patients for over twenty years without a single adverse report. I have taken them myself for even longer than that and am still fit and well in spite of my own arthritis, which hardly ever inconveniences me.

GLANDULAR. The commonest of this group is ovarian deficiency which is easily diagnosed by the menstrual history. It may take the form of irregular or painful periods, with two to five days of pre-menstrual depression and backache. The backache is most likely to be an exacerbation of a rheumatic condition which, so far, may not have been bad enough for the patient to seek advice and will certainly not be diagnosed as such. The symptoms subside with the onset of menstruation and are forgotten about, in mild cases, until the next cycle. Even where a doctor has been consulted, medication with pain-killers is the usual story. In established cases of arthritis the symptoms are always worse before the period starts. It is surprising how often the patients themselves do not realize this until it has been pointed out to them.

I have found that almost every female patient gains weight up to 2–3 lbs (about one kilo) in the two or three days before the period starts. This is due to not passing the normal amount of urine, which leaves excess fluid in the body, giving rise to a feeling of heaviness and depression plus increased pain and discomfort. This can be treated on a temporary basis by taking a water-reducing pill. The real treatment, however, is to correct the failure of the ovaries (by giving an appropriate ovarian preparation such as Diphaston at the proper time, so that the period becomes normal).

The importance of treating this glandular disturbance is not only to relieve the symptoms of pain and depression but because the function of the ovary is an integral part of the whole body-mechanism. Without it, it is like expecting a Rolls Royce to behave perfectly when one of its cylinders is cracked.

The improvement of rheumatoid arthritis cases by dealing with this aspect of the disease has been quite significant. Further evidence of this beneficial effect can be seen in those women who have experienced a great improvement in their rheumatic symptoms during pregnancy, when the cycle of ovarian function was not necessary.

When women approach the menopause (change of life) around about fifty, there develops a natural decline in the function of the ovaries. Some patients suffer a severe disturbance which frequently aggravates a mild rheumatic condition, so that these symptoms become much worse and a hitherto mild arthritic condition becomes more active. This is the type of arthritis which doctors call 'menopausal arthritis', but, of course, it has been there in most cases for at least twenty years! Treating the severe flushes and depression with a different form of ovarian hormone will always mitigate the symptoms and help to improve the arthritis. It should, however, be clearly understood that the change of life is a natural development, and the use of a hormone should be used with discrimination. In principle, I believe it to be wrong to interfere with natural development or regression unless there is good evidence that it is abnormal. Once the change of life is over, the arthritis tends to settle down.

OCCUPATIONAL. The problem of the strain of work and travelling is too obvious to need much discussion. The work-load applies with equal force to the mother at home with its endless demands on her limited health. It is unfair to expect any treatment to be really successful unless the body is given adequate rest during the active stages of the illness.

ENVIRONMENTAL. Here again the problems of damp and bad housing, an unhappy household and financial strain do not require anything more than a mere statement of fact to be considered in the pattern of treatment if it is to be successful.

PSYCHOLOGICAL. The psychological factor has two important aspects. Firstly, rheumatism may occur in an individual who is primarily disturbed psychologically from other causes, either physical or induced by unhappy or misguided family problems. It is important to appreciate this type, because the rheumatic condition may be very minor and merely used as a means of obtaining sympathy. I believe this kind of case is rare. The genuine rheumatic case with an anxiety overlay is very real. Part of the depression is certainly due to the illness, with its tiredness, aching and inability to cope with the physical demands, either at school or work. It may even be aggravated by ill-advised treatment.

The anxiety overlay which gives it the 'psychological aspect' is, in no small measure, due to the fact that doctors do not recognize the condition and therefore tend to think the patient is either imagining or overstressing symptoms. This is the time when tranquillizers are prescribed. By dulling the patient's sensitivity to pain and thought, the tranquillizers act as a crutch for the patient and a prop for the doctor. What a parody of real medicine, worthy of Gilbert and Sullivan treatment! Do not think for one moment that I am exaggerating. During the last ten years almost every patient who has consulted me was taking tranquillizers in addition to all the other rheumatic drugs. Here is a quotation from a report by Dr W. A. R. Thomson in the *Daily Telegraph*, of some doctors in Ipswich who laudably have eradicated the prescribing of barbiturates from their practice: "Patients complaining of backache, stiff neck and the like, walk out of their doctors' surgeries with a prescription of the latest tranquillizers."

There is a further aspect of the anxiety felt by many patients who see no real progress in their own cases and get depressed at seeing so many older cases, whom they meet in hospital waiting-rooms, continuing to deteriorate in spite of treatment.

6

Specific Treatment—Group A

VIRUS INFECTION. Because all the early symptoms of rheumatism so closely resemble a muted form of influenza, and because many rheumatic symptoms develop after an attack of influenza, the clinical justification for using an influenza-virus vaccine cannot be denied. You will see evidence as to its value in some of the cases detailed later, but first let me tell you about myself.

I contracted my first attack of influenza in the terrible epidemic of 1934–5. It was the one which killed thousands of patients and left many who recovered with suicidal tendencies, some of whom succeeded in achieving their aim with gas ovens or by jumping off bridges.

I lost over a stone in weight and took seven weeks to recover. On my first week back at work I woke up in the middle of the night with a terrible pain in the upper part of my back. By the morning I realized I had my first attack of rheumatism. Although I did not like the pain, I was greatly intrigued by it. It introduced me in a very practical manner to the pain about which so many of my patients came to consult me! Perhaps it made me more keen to solve the problem. Since that first attack of influenza, I very rarely went more than one year without another bout. My medical history thereafter was strewn with attacks of influenza and repeated attacks of rheumatism which affected my neck, all parts of my back and particularly my hands.

Around 1954, when influenza vaccines made their *début*, I was a very eager candidate. Since that time I have not had a single attack of influenza, and consequently my rheumatism has not been subject to its annual aggravation. I have so much arthritis in my spine and yet so little pain. Much credit for keeping free from influenza must go to the vaccine, although I have no doubt of the value of the other method of treatment for rheumatism. My hands in particular show very little evidence of what I suffered years ago.

Because no virus has been found in any arthritic joint— that is the only place in which they have been sought, it does not mean that a virus is not to be found elsewhere. You will recall that I have demonstrated beyond any reasonable doubt that the rheumatic patch is the first localized manifestation of the disease during or immediately following all those symptoms of ill-health described earlier in the text. If a virus is responsible for these symptoms, then we are more likely to find it in the early stages of a rheumatic patch than at any other time or place. The enormous problem of their identification is created because, during their activity in attacking the cells, they appear to become merged in the destruction of those very cells—rather like Samson when he brought down the Temple.

Perhaps it may best be illustrated by picturing the live virus as a lighted match which starts a fire. The fire eventually destroys both the match and all the materials it has set alight, so that all that is left are ash and charred remains at the periphery. It may be impossible at this stage to distinguish between the ashes of the virus and the tissues which have been attacked. It is equally unlikely that you could revitalize them in the laboratory for the purposes of identification. If, however, you could be present at the onset of the fire, then you would have a much greater chance of identifying the cause of it. As I have indicated before, investigation of the joints is like poking around in the charred periphery, whereas we are likely to find the virus only if we investigate the rheumatic patches in the very early stages, which may be a matter of only a day or two before the virus becomes part of the ash.

I am glad to be able to report that I have been extremely fortunate, through the good offices of Dr Freed, in enlisting the active interest and participation of the clinical research unit Northwick Park which is presently engaged in studying these rheumatic patches for the evidence of a virus or specific damage to the tissues which might be viral in origin.

In many cases I believe it might be the actual influenza virus which causes the rheumatism. The influenza-virus strains vary from time to time, and there must surely be some varieties which can cause rheumatism. My experience suggests that immunization with the influenza virus may be specific in some cases, but where it is not, stimulating antibody reaction to it may help against other strains. These vaccines should be given to the patients when they are well, in a period of remission and preferably with an initial dose which is smaller than that recommended.

DIPHTHEROID VACCINE. I developed this form of treatment between 1947 and 1950. This is the story of how it came about.

I joined the staff of the Charterhouse Rheumatism Clinic in 1937. The standard treatment for every patient attending the clinic was a weekly injection of vaccine which was made up from a combination of six bacteria which Dr Warren Grove, the founder of the clinic, had isolated and cultured from the throats of hundreds of arthritis patients. The theory that arthritis was caused by infection was frequently discussed and investigated at that time all over the world, and many forms of vaccine were produced, particularly in America. After some time, I remained quite unconvinced that the vaccines at the Charterhouse Rheumatism Clinic were of any demonstrable value.

I studied a very long series of throat-swab reports at the clinic to see if there was any combination or permutation of the six main suspected bacteria which might throw a new angle on the problem. Nothing at all emerged from this until one day it struck me that there was one very common bacteria which hardly ever appeared. This was the diphtheroid organism. I studied the history of these germs back through fifty years of recorded medical and scientific reports. No, it could not be incriminated as a disease-causing germ. I then got the idea (which today is glorified with the description of 'lateral thinking') that maybe the patients were not so well because the diphtheroid germs were driven out of their normal habitat and other, more pathological germs, had taken their place. The idea that some germs were favourable to mankind was now being accepted. For example, there was one called 'bac. proteus' which is known to facilitate the formation of vitamin K; there are others without which the bowel cannot remain healthy. On this assumption, I decided to try the effect of an injection made up of two strains of diphtheroid germs. It is, strictly speaking, not a vaccine. A vaccine, like the influenza vaccine, for example, works by giving small doses of dead or nearly dead germs in order to stimulate the body's reaction to those germs, so that by the time the real germ arrives, the patient would be in a prepared condition to resist. The diphtheroid preparation was given in the hope that it introduced into the body something which might be beneficial. The patients were given a weekly injection of the diphtheroids. All the details of an exhaustive investigation and trials were published in an article in the official journal *Rheumatism* of the Charterhouse Rheumatism Clinic in 1950. The results, with an improvement rate of 92 per cent, fully justified the use of this vaccine, and I have been using it ever since.

What is now quite remarkable, indeed very exciting for me, is that in 1979 Dr Georges E. Werner, in the Department of Virology and Immunology at a research unit in France, published a scientific article in which he proved that the diphtheroid organisms protected animals from the severe and often fatal results of various strains of virus, with which they were inoculated after first being injected with the diphtheroids. Towards the end of his report he states that it does not appear that clinical studies have been performed (this means on human beings) to demonstrate a beneficial effect of this agent in diseases caused by viruses. I could not wish for better or more independent evidence than his to support my theory formulated over thirty years ago. It surely must help to sustain my claims of its beneficial effect in the rheumatic diseases. Of course, he could not have been aware of my work with the very high percentage-rate of success. This may very well be due to the passage of time, together with the insuperable obstacles to my efforts in getting the work publicized.

During all these years there has never been a single case of any adverse reaction and I continue to be encouraged by its beneficial effect. I may add that the Warren Crowe vaccine, along with all the others, have long since been abandoned.

Because of the failure of all these other forms of vaccines, the idea that arthritis was not infective in nature began to gain ground. In fact, all that had been proved was that those suspected organisms were not the cause of the rheumatism, but it did not prove that there was no infection. The general tendency was then to doubt the theory of infection, which it seems still has some adherents in the profession. To discard the theory of infection is to deny all the basic medical teachings of clinical medicine upon which all past successes have been built. There has never been any recognizable disease, associated with a rise of temperature, for which bacteria or virus has not been identified at some stage since scientific technology had made it possible. Why should arthritis be any different? I have already established that a rise in temperature occurs in the early stages of the disease and also during the periods of relapse.

Because the disease is not recognized by the rheumatism specialists until X-ray evidence is positive, they have missed all the early clinical signs which I have described in my book. The lack of this clinical understanding is the basic reason why the solution of this terrible disease continues to elude them.

What now remains to be discussed is the treatment of the rheumatic patches and the use of anti-rheumatic drugs.

RHEUMATIC PATCHES. These are injected locally with a

special solution of sodium salicylate which I have devised. It is really a salt of aspirin, and it seemed a good idea to place some in an affected area in a concentration which could never be achieved by taking aspirin by mouth.

The interesting point about the injection is that it is completely painless in healthy tissue but very painful in the rheumatic patch. Fortunately, the pain never lasts for more than sixty seconds and is followed by almost immediate relief of the symptoms. The pain caused by the injection is a safeguard for both the patient and the doctor. If there is no pain on injection, there will be no improvement—you have missed the patch. In practice, no patient likes the pain, but they are more than willing to submit because of the improvement which so rapidly follows.

In those cases where the patches are localized in only one or two areas and the disease is not in an active state, this treatment may be all that is required to bring about an early and astonishing improvement in the symptoms. This has happened in cases of stiff necks, tennis elbow, wrist and knee. The hip is often more difficult because there are usually very many patches, some deep-seated, and the arthritis is usually much more advanced because of weight-bearing. I have had successes, but they do take much longer.

Where the disease is active, the inflammation tends to extend, and even though you may help a local patch, you cannot stop the spread of the inflammation with the local injection. This can be achieved only by improving the patient's resistance by the measures already outlined. During this period the use of anti-rheumatic drugs and pain-relievers may be justified. It must be clearly understood, however, that not one of these drugs can cure the disease, be it rheumatoid arthritis or osteo-arthritis. It is naïve of doctors to believe that any of the so-called anti-inflammatory drugs are in any way curative, and it is totally wrong for the patient to be given false hopes.

There has been an endless stream of these drugs since the discovery of cortisone, all trying to reproduce its good effects and minimize its bad effects. The evils of cortisone have long been demonstrated, but there is still a lack of recognition by the profession that cortisone produced 'success' by masking the symptoms of pain, thus allowing the patient to use the limbs normally, whilst the disease itself continued to cause more and more damage to the joint. Even with the small doses used today to relieve symptoms, the same principle of non-cure obtains.

What all these new drugs do and how they work is still not really understood. As they are produced, so they replace the older ones, simply because time has demonstrated the relative futility of those gone before. None of these drugs can really show any substantial advance on aspirin, which is the only one I use. This does not mean that my patients take it regularly—not at all, only if they have a relapse and then only for a few days at the most. Occasionally, if a patient has a relapse with generalized pain and is intolerant to aspirin, butozolidine gives quite a dramatic relief within twenty-four hours. Only in such cases should it be used until the attack is over. If that immediate response is absent, it is no use trying again—it will not work, and unpleasant side-effects may occur. There are now enough preparations of aspirin to overcome most of its unpleasant effects to allow most people to use it as and when required, not the constant and interminable repetition of all those other drugs.

It must be stressed that I use aspirin in this restricted way just to relieve the symptoms and make the patient more comfortable, not because there is any proof of its curative powers.

The principle which has ever been my guide is that all drugs are poisonous to a greater or lesser degree, so that they should be used only when their good effects outweigh the bad ones. That is why I am completely bemused by the widespread use of so many pain-killing drugs and the multiplicity of anti-inflammatory drugs, which my patients never seem to need. So many of them have told me how they resented the continual drugging they have been subjected to, for so little, if any, improvement. As I pointed out earlier, they do not know enough to be able to question their doctor's treatment.

Now let me give you a few examples of cases I have

treated. This will enable you to see how the treatment works and how it can be applied to your own case.

Case 1
Rheumatoid Arthritis—Mrs M. S. aged 41

This patient complained of constant pain in both hips, ten years in the right hip and the last five in the left one, which was now more painful than the right. She was rarely free from pain but obtained some relief when resting. She could take only short steps and could not keep up with her companions when walking to a bus or subway.

All her symptoms got much worse for one week before her period started and were accompanied by that dreadful depression so many ladies experience at that time. She could recall very severe attacks of influenza in 1960 and 1970, both of which could be related to a worsening of her arthritis. She had had a stiff back most of her life and could remember a severe attack of rheumatism affecting both her hands in 1957 and pain in the right hip at the age of ten. She nursed her mother, who had rheumatoid arthritis for many years, which accounted for a late and childless marriage.

She had been diagnosed and treated in hospital, but her condition was slowly and relentlessly worsening. That is why she came to see me. At the first consultation I injected some rheumatic patches in her back which immediately improved the left hip, and she was able to walk better. For three weeks she had vitamin and local rheumatic-patch injections, three times a week, and a diphtheroid injection once weekly, by which time she was able to walk much better, had much less pain and felt much better. The only drug she took was the anti-histamine I prescribed—Phenergan 10 mgs at night. I also treated her menstrual disorder with injections of progesterone (this can now be done with tablets). After the first three weeks, treatment was gradually reduced to once weekly, and within five months she was vastly improved, had no pain, could take almost full strides and had no more period pain or depression.

The important point to remember is that the disease for

those last few years was localized to the lower back and both hips, so recovery was rapid.

Case 2
Rheumatoid Arthritis—Mrs E. R. S. aged 63

The third finger of her left hand and the fifth finger of her right hand were swollen, cold and very painful, the left for four months and the right for two months. She could not use either finger, whilst both hands were always painful on movement, and she suffered a constant nag. She had to wear splints to support her wrists. In 1961 her right fourth finger had to be amputated for a similar condition. In 1970 her left fourth finger was amputated. Ever since she had experienced phantom pain in both absent fingers.

She came to me as a last resort before going back for further amputations. Her general condition was very poor, and no wonder. I gave her intensive vitamin treatment, diphtheroid vaccine, anti-histamines Benadryl and Ephedrine, and injections in rheumatic patches in her arm.

The improvement in her fingers within four days was dramatic. After three weeks her fingers were normal, her phantom pains were abolished, and her splints were thrown away. Her treatment followed the usual pattern of increased intervals between visits. For almost two years she had no treatment and is happily working and playing the piano. In this case the remarkably quick recovery was made possible because the disease was localized to both hands.

Case 3
Rheumatoid Arthritis—Mr H. B. aged 47

This man was a newsagent and confectioner. Eighteen months before he consulted me, he had tripped over a rope. Some weeks later he developed a pain in the right knee, and both his hands became swollen and painful. The hands seemed to settle down after one week, but the knee became much worse, followed by pain and swelling in the other knee and both ankles. He was very stiff in the morning and after sitting during the day. He was unable to walk without a stick. Later, some of his fingers became swollen and painful. He had been treated in hospital, but nothing they did could stop the remorseless progression of the disease.

I injected some rheumatic patches related to the left knee in order to show him that it was possible to improve the condition and to give him hope for the future. I warned him that the condition was active—note how it was spreading from one knee to so many other joints. It was essential to improve his general health and to build up his resistance. I gave the usual treatment of vitamins, diphtheroid injections, anti-histamines and aspirin as a temporary measure, and an occasional injection of Butozolidine when there was a flare-up.

He made gradual and continuous progress, with, of course, treatment sessions decreasing to once in two weeks. After five months he was so well that I suspended all treatment with an injunction to return as soon as any trouble started. He did have relapses, which were always preceded by mild influenzal symptoms, sore throat or bronchitis. Recovery was always rapid, and as the influenza vaccine began to improve his resistance, so the attacks disappeared, and he has remained fit ever since. The only 'treatment' he has needed is the influenza vaccine every six months and an anti-histamine at night.

The point to remember about this patient is that the disease was very active, and the success of the treatment depended more on general treatment to improve resistance and less on the injection of the rheumatic patches.

A further point of interest is that no marked trouble started in his knee until about three weeks after tripping over a rope. If the fall had been bad enough to cause injury to the knee, he should have felt it immediately—but he did not. The answer to that was that his knee let him down, and he thought he had tripped, when in fact his first rheumatic patch had appeared in that area. He had one of those 'sprains' I described earlier in the book.

Case 4
Rheumatoid Arthritis—Mrs J. M. B. aged 58
This patient had had aching in her back and both legs for

two years. The right knee was painful and swollen for one year, and the left knee started to be painful one month previously. She also had twinges of pain in her right shoulder and the fingers of her right hand for six months. Pains woke her up at night. There was a history of dermatitis, and she had lost 21 pounds in weight.

The usual treatment was instituted, and within two weeks improvement was well on the way. In a period of two years she had five relapses which all rapidly responded to rest and treatment. Since then she has been free of all symptoms.

The main reason for quoting this case is that this patient had two sisters with rheumatoid arthritis. The younger sister, aged fifty-six, started when she was fourteen and up to date had had both hip joints and both knee joints replaced, with satisfactory results. The other sister started at the age of forty-seven in exactly the same way as my patient. The deterioration was persistent, and within ten years both knee joints had to be replaced. The downward trend of my patient has so far been reversed. She has no swelling of the knees and is able to live a full and normal life. I am confident that, providing she returns for treatment on relapse, she can expect never to become crippled. Note also the clear evidence of allergy—the dermatitis.

Case 5
Frozen Shoulder—Mrs S. P. aged 47

First consultation 14th September 1970. The patient complained of persistent pain in the right upper arm often extending down to her fingers—not a single day free from pain in last nine months. It started as a frozen shoulder eight years ago, and she had had very little relief during the whole time. Pain often woke her up at night. In the last three months she had developed pain in left thigh. Previous treatment in hospital and privately included physiotherapy, manipulation and an assortment of drugs; the only one which gave her any relief was Panadol. She felt ill and depressed although normally was of a carefree nature. She had a history of sore throats and some allergy, presenting as mild, infrequent dermatitis and headaches following even a sip or two of wine.

Treatment followed: the usual pattern of vitamins, diphtheroid vaccine, anti-histamine and aspirin. I treated rheumatic patches in the leg first as it was so recent, and this responded very quickly. The shoulder problem of eight years' duration took some time, but there was continual improvement after each treatment. She had full use of her arm within three months. There were the usual relapses, mostly heralded by generalized aching, just as one gets with influenza. They always responded to rest and aspirin, in addition to the diphtheroid vaccine. In due course, she kept well with six-monthly influenza vaccine and of course always taking the anti-histamine.

After eight years of pain, disability and drug-taking, she is pain-free with full movement of her arm and leg.

Case 6
Osteo-Arthritis (Hip)—Mrs S. M. aged 46

This patient complained of worsening pain and stiffness in the left leg for twelve years. She had great difficulty in putting on shoes and stockings and in going up and down stairs and was unable to mount a horse for a very long time. (She had a riding-school.) No treatment had helped her, and she was told that a replacement of the hip would have to be done in a year or two. She had all the symptoms of a generalized active rheumatic condition, with generalized aching, sweating and sore throats. She was also under-going the menopausal changes.

Treatment of a deep rheumatic patch in the back gave immediate relief to the hip trouble. I often do this for a patient at the first consultation, just to demonstrate that there is hope, even though I stress that no permanent improvement can be expected until they have developed some resistance to the disease. Apart from the usual treatment, I added a small dose of a hormone to reduce the severe change-of-life symptoms.

Within four or five weeks she was walking much better, had no trouble going up and down the staircase and was even able to mount a horse again, although she wisely decided not to ride any more. Of course, there were relapses in her condition because all the general symptoms returned from time to time, but in spite of this the hip managed to retain its progress.

This case demonstrates quite clearly the general infective nature of the illness which expressed itself mainly in the hip. The worsening of her condition also coincided with the menopause, which I dealt with earlier. However, although the disease is being contained, there is a failure to develop a resistance to it, which accounts for the relapses.

Case 7
Non-Articular—Mr D. E. aged 38

I first attended this patient for pains in the legs in 1950 when he was fourteen years old. I diagnosed him then as a rheumatic case and so advised his mother. I also recommended his headmaster not to push him at physical exercises and games and to make allowances for his tiredness which he suspected was laziness. As a result, he got through school with a minimum of discomfort.

At the age of eighteen he was working as an electrical assistant when he developed aches and pains in both thighs, which improved with rest and worsened after walking. He also had cramp in his legs at night, and his eyesight became weaker, for which he was prescribed glasses. From then on he had recurrent attacks of aching and pain affecting almost every part of his body. He had married, had two children and because of ill-health had financial problems and all the strain that goes with them.

He visited me only rarely because he lived so far away and relied on his local doctor and hospital. He was a frequent visitor to hospital, and in spite of my medical report he was investigated at a Neurological Centre in 1965 where the diagnosis was "Low back pain, rt. sciatica, spinabifida S.1 Marfans syndrome and possible non-infective Addisonian syndrome." Here is a long list of illnesses in this patient arrived at by the application of modern scientific medicine—enough to daunt the general practitioner, the patient and all lay people—he must be pretty lucky to be alive! When the list is analysed, low back pain and sciatica are merely facets of his rheumatic condition, a word not mentioned in the diagnosis; the 'spinabifida' he was born with had never caused him any trouble in his early years, so why now? Marfans syndrome is an abstruse condition recently invented and has no relevance to his illness; the Addisonian syndrome is only a possibility. The sum of all these investigations left the patient in precisely the same state as before.

Since then he has never been fit, always has pain somewhere, spends more time being ill than working and is often in hospital.

In May 1973 I treated his back on two occasions which gave him some relief, and again in November with an even better result. He returned in March 1974 with severe pain in his right hip, leg and neck. All the standard treatment was used regularly. He made a good recovery and was discharged in May 1974, looking very well and feeling well, in spite of the earlier scientific diagnosis. His was a long, sad history, most of which could have been avoided if he could have rested and had the right treatment when attacks came on. All his hospital stays and treatment were of no avail. He is still a young man, of impeccable character, who could be helped enormously by being given the right kind of sedentary occupation with an adequate salary to support his family. This is a case where the occupational and environmental factors are as important to a recovery as the correct medical treatment, which, unfortunately, he got only when he came to see me.

Case 8
Non-Articular—Mr H. W. aged 47
There was a long history of aches and pains since the second decade, and always associated with tiredness. He had had attacks in hands, arms, back, legs and in his earlier years was in hospital for six months for pain in the left hip. Many of his attacks had been accompanied by temperature and sweating, which necessitated bed-rest for short periods.

Sodium salicylate seemed the most effective drug. He is very sensitive to drugs, even Phenergan made him drowsy, but he does manage 15 mgs. Ephedrine. Lately his pains have become more localized, particularly in the upper back.

The pains always respond to rest and are relieved with Butozolidine, but recurrences are frequent.

He has had all the standard treatments, but I must rate him as one of my most disappointing cases. The clinical history is so clearly an infective one that I believe he must be a case where special investigation for a virus might prove valuable.

The lessons to be learned from these cases are that patients can be greatly helped without the need for endless drug-taking, either to relieve pain or to induce sleep. Heat, massage and physiotherapy are mostly superfluous, and, as I have pointed out, massage can actually be harmful.

I have included Case 8 in order to show that there are cases which defy treatment simply because they cannot develop an immunity to the disease and will have to wait until the virus has been isolated. It should act as a warning that not everybody can expect to be helped at this time.

How can you apply all this advice to your own case? What can you do to get this treatment? Let us start with what you can do for yourself:

1. Whenever you get a sore throat, influenza, laryngitis or bronchitis, insist on 24–48 hours' rest. Take aspirin three or four times a day. Remember, two days' rest at this time will probably save weeks of misery later.
2. Whenever the disease begins to intensify (you get general achiness, more tiredness, increased pain in some already affected areas), rest and take aspirin as required. If you have a temperature—it may be only very slight $\frac{1}{2}$–1°F, spend more time in bed, otherwise just resting in an armchair, reading or watching the television, is enough.
3. Any part of your body which suddenly gets worse should be rested. Remember, it is all due to inflammation, the basic medical treatment for which is rest.
4. A small dose of anti-histamine should be taken one hour before going to bed.
5. Get out of your mind the idea that you will stiffen up if you do not keep moving—you will not.
6. Do not accept any form of massage or exercise until you know that the disease is not in an active state—that is,

when your disability is restricted to localized pain and some stiffness. There must be no general aching, severe tiredness or temperature.

7. Wean yourself off all other drugs. You may feel worse for a while due to withdrawal symptoms, but you will soon get over it, and maybe you can dispense with sleeping-pills in due course.

8. Eat a good varied diet and get some extra vitamins, particularly B and C, from your doctor, instead of drugs.

Influenza vaccine, diphtheroid injections and local aspirin injections are treatments which can be given only by a doctor. I am sure that when the profession as a whole is made aware of the need and value of this new approach, they will be only too anxious to co-operate.

7

Allied Diseases—Groups B and C

In the previous chapter I dealt with the treatment of rheumatic cases which would be clearly recognized as such by everybody, including the medical profession. I am now going to describe cases which are given various medical names but which are really rheumatic conditions and should be treated in the same way.

The late Professor Sir William Osler (there is still a medical society justifiably dedicated to his clinical wisdom) wrote, in his celebrated work on medicine, that no doctor should ever consider himself adequately equipped in diagnosis unless he fully understood syphilis. He rightly claimed that the disease, because of its long-drawn-out character and ramifications throughout the whole body, could mimic almost every known disease. There is no doubt at all in my mind that was entirely true in his time. Nowadays, it is rheumatism which is even more widespread than syphilis ever was and actually mimics far more diseases. I will demonstrate the truth of this claim with the following examples:

MIGRAINE
This word is used to cover any sort of recurrent headache.

You need only to read the pamphlet of the Migraine Trust to see what I mean. Of course, it would exclude headaches for which a cause could be found, such as bad eyesight, brain disorder or sinus disease.

I have treated many cases where recurrent headache was one of the symptoms of the rheumatic complaint, but I did not call them migraine. To me they were just part of the rheumatic disease process. The headache was a pain felt in some part of the head and caused by a rheumatic patch in exactly the same way as a sprain in the wrist or ankle. However, I have treated a number of migraine cases. Let me tell you about two of the earliest ones:

Mrs C. C. aged 26
This patient consulted me in May 1968 for pain in the right hip. This was a rheumatic condition which I treated and which soon got better.

Some time after that, her husband consulted me about some pains in his back which were also rheumatic and which I was able to cure. In the course of conversation he told me that his wife suffered from severe migraine attacks, associated with vomiting and lasting for about twenty-four hours. They never knew when the attack would occur, and frequently they had to cancel appointments at very short notice. She had seen several specialists, both here and in America, without success.

It is interesting to note that she did not even mention them to me when she first consulted me about her hip. This was due to the quite common belief that migraine is a special illness for which you must have a specialist. Accordingly, she thought that, as the migraine specialist she had already seen did not help, there would seem to be no point in telling a rheumatologist. Very soon after, she came to see me, and I found rheumatic patches in her neck. After three injections with sodium salicylate into these patches, she was completely cured. She needed no more drugs except a small dose of Benadryl (an anti-histamine), as a precaution which, as you know, I consider invaluable in most rheumatic cases.

Mrs D.B. aged 36

She had attacks at intervals of one month. They lasted up to four days each and were so severe that she had to stay in a darkened room most of the time. There was persistent vomiting, and she had to take a lot of drugs. Her first attack was at the age of ten. For many years she had about four to five attacks per year, but in the last seven years these had become more frequent, i.e. one every month.

I found rheumatic patches in her neck. Treatment of these patches produced immediate improvement. After the first salicylate injection she said her head felt clearer than she could ever remember. She had nine injections in three weeks, and then gradually these were reduced. After two months she did not need any more injections and was free from all her previous misery. Again, the only drug I recommended was a mild anti-histamine.

During the last two years I have successfully treated four more cases. Therefore, in the cases of severe migraine I can claim a 100 per cent cure. Is this luck, coincidence or correct diagnosis and treatment? I do not claim and in fact do not know whether every case of migraine has rheumatic patches, but I do know that the patients I have treated had them. I have no doubt that many migraine sufferers have them.

Here is an example of another form of neck trouble:

Mr F. G. aged 40

I first saw him in February 1967. He had continuous pain and stiffness in his neck for five months. He had received all the usual treatment, including heat, massage, manipulation and traction. His pains became worse, and I have no doubt that the treatment contributed to it. Finally, he was put into a collar. The pain continued and the collar was very uncomfortable.

At this stage he consulted me. I found the usual rheumatic patches—two superficial and two deep. After the first local injection he was immediately improved and discarded the collar, with great relief. After three treatments he was almost normal. He had slight relapse in April which required three more treatments, and he has remained free ever since.

In retrospect, I realized that the cause of the relapse was due to my not dealing with the rheumatic patches adequately. After all, I was still learning a great deal about them!

Moving down the body from the head and neck to the chest, take the case of a man, about fifty years old. He gets a sudden pain in the chest over the heart area. He does not know what it is, but it is frightening. Even if he is the stolid type, his wife or children may be very concerned. There are always the relatives or friends who know somebody who had a pain like that, who either died of a heart attack or was saved by immediate removal to the Intensive Care Unit of the hospital. The stage is now set for the great DRAMA and the arrival of the doctor. He does an examination and says, "Well, it might be—I am not sure, we had better have a heart specialist." The specialist duly arrives, or the patient is sent to hospital. He has an electrocardiogram if at home, X-rays and blood-tests in addition if he goes into hospital. He has either had a heart attack or not. If he has, then all this effort is justifiable and correct. What if he has not had a heart attack? The pain perhaps goes, and he is so relieved that he does not think to ask what it was. He may be told it was just a strain, or something else equally unintelligible.

I believe any doctor worth his keep should be able to judge very quickly whether there has been a heart attack or not. 99 per cent of patients with a heart attack show unmistakable signs, in their face, breathing, pulse and heartbeat. I therefore doubt very much that a positive diagnosis will ever be missed.

Why, then, do so many cases occur where the doctors are not sure? The answer is quite clear: they cannot think of an alternative diagnosis. They are not aware that the pain may have been caused by a rheumatic patch between the ribs, over the heart or near the spine, involving the nerve going round the chest at the same level. In this case it is the sudden occurrence of a rheumatic patch which causes the pain, and it is likely to get better in a day or two, just as I explained to you in an earlier chapter.

I am quite certain that if doctors knew about and understood these rheumatic patches, they would so easily be able to say with confidence, "No, you have not had a heart attack—it is a bit of rheumatism which we can soon put right." Imagine how many false alarms would be scotched—how much less anxiety would be generated and how much manpower and money would be saved, by not requiring the visit of a specialist, an ambulance to hospital and all the unnecessary investigation.

What I have said about heart attacks is bad enough, but what now of angina? This is a condition which nearly always is present for some time before a heart attack. Its main symptoms are pain on exertion and breathlessness. This diagnosis should never be in doubt, but read what Dr M. H. Pappworth had to say in his article 'Diagnosing Angina Pectoris' in *World Medicine*, 17th May 1978: "Genuine angina is rarely missed but is often wrongly suspected or even definitely diagnosed when it is not present—a serious error often made not only by GPs but by hospital doctors at all levels of seniority. Some doctors are afraid of not labelling anybody with chest pain as having angina lest they be proved wrong"—when they get a heart attack. The whole of his article not only confirms what I claim about wrong diagnosis and treatment, but the tenor of his criticism is more strongly worded than mine. Following on this, he describes a number of cases where the diagnosis was wrong and gives very precise details of signs and symptoms which should enable every doctor to know for certain if it is a true case of angina or not. Unfortunately, he is not able to offer an alternative diagnosis, excepting vague suggestion of other structures in the body being affected—by what? I have no doubt at all that, were he aware of the rheumatic patch, he would frequently find the real answer to false angina. How better to convince a patient and a perplexed doctor that you have a demonstrable alternative diagnosis which is capable of immediate proof and successful treatment?

Let me quote the case of Mr F., aged forty, from NE Region. He consulted me because of what I had done for his daughter, Susan F., aged nine, a case dealt with a little later.

He developed a sudden pain in his chest, with breathlessness and shallow breathing. He was taken to hospital, where the whole routine for angina and heart attack was gone through. There was no electrocardiographic evidence of disease, but he was treated on the same basis as if he had—just as Dr Pappworth describes. As he was making no progress and was very worried, he decided to consult me. He had a persistent pain in the left side of his chest which caused him difficulty in breathing normally. I confirmed that his heart and pulse were normal, but I did find a rheumatic patch on the left side of the spine. This I injected, and immediately the pain was relieved and his breathing became much easier. No heart attack, no angina and now no symptoms, so no anxiety. There was no further trouble after that. This case illustrates the fact that it is not much use to a patient if you assure him he has not got angina but cannot relieve his symptoms.

The chest pains may occur on the other side, or below the heart level on either side, so that the question now will be, are the lungs affected? If the patch affects a muscle between the ribs, then it will make breathing painful whenever that particular muscle has to play its part. The result is that the patient tends to avoid using that muscle, and so the breathing becomes shallower and shorter. That causes anxiety in the patient's mind and so aggravates the condition. Once again, the doctor is not sure whether there is 'a touch of pleurisy' or even something more serious. Once again, all the paraphernalia of investigation is brought into action, and like many of the suspected heart cases, some of these patients end up in hospital. I repeat, the general practitioners can hardly be blamed for their indecision because they have never heard of these patches, and without an alternative diagnosis, what can they do but protect the patient and themselves?

In the abdomen there are many organs that can be subject to disease and so cause pain, which is the overriding reason for people consulting their doctor. It is sometimes easy for the doctor to decide what the cause of pain is: for example, gall-stones, kidney-stones, gastric ulcer, colitis. Sometimes these cases are not so easily determined, but a definite diagnosis can usually be established by a detailed examination and X-rays. Remember, these are the cases of major illnesses which should present no real problem to your local doctor. Now let us consider the cases where the patient has a nagging indeterminate pain or ache in the abdominal area. It comes and goes, does not seem to have any real relationship to eating or drinking, and sometimes disappears altogether for no obvious reason; equally, it reappears without any reason. There is really nothing you can tell the doctor which will help to locate the trouble to any particular organ. After trying various remedies, or even before, you will be sent to hospital for investigation. In these types of cases, nothing will be found, so it will not be long before you become an object of suspicion, just as I have already described.

To be fair, there are some specialists who do realize the inadequacy of medical knowledge. They are not afraid to say "I do not know" and do not suspect the patient of neurosis. Some years ago a surgeon, Mr Daintree Johnson of the Royal Free Hospital, wrote a letter to the *Lancet* expressing those sentiments. More recently, in July 1977, The *British Medical Journal* printed an article on undiagnosed abdominal pain, which contained this statement: "Without doubt, undiagnosed abdominal pain is a common and frustrating problem which merits more detailed investigation." Most cases were subjected to laparotomy—that is the name given to opening up the abdomen in order to see what might be wrong. In some they found cancer and other diseases, but in others they found nothing. Had they known about the rheumatic patch, it might have saved quite a number from the operation. Let me give two examples:

Mrs K. G. aged 28
3rd March 1971: she complains of constant aching in the lower chest area, various parts of the abdomen and the back. It all started after her baby was born eighteen months previously. She is never free from pain and feels ill and depressed; her mother has to look after the baby. She has a hairdressing business with which she can hardly cope. She

has been extensively investigated, including X-rays of gall-bladder, kidneys, stomach and bowel. When her mother had to return to her home in Cyprus, the patient was so ill that she agreed to let her mother take the baby with her.

The clue to all her troubles was the rheumatic patches I found in her back. The disease was very active. With rest and intensive treatment she was soon improved and by July was free from all symptoms and able to have her baby back.

Susan F. aged 9
She is Mr F.'s daughter, referred to earlier, a sweet little girl who had a pain in her stomach on the left side for two months; she never had a single day without pain. She also developed constipation at the same time, for which she was given laxatives. The pain was always worse at school when sitting at her desk. It did not seem to bother her when walking or playing.

She was sent to a teaching hospital, where investigations proved negative. No diagnosis or treatment was given, and she was asked to report back in two months' time. She was missing quite a lot of schooling, and it did look a bit suspicious. Her parents believed her, however, and brought her to see me.

The clue to her trouble was that the pain came on and worsened when she was bending over her schoolbook on the desk or when she was in a similar position at the table at home. I soon discovered the rheumatic patch in her back. It required only two injections to cure her pain completely. The laxatives were stopped, and with a little training, her bowel movements became normal.

So far, the rheumatic patches I have discussed occur in the neck or as far down as the twelfth dorsal vertebra which you can see on the diagram. The nerves which come out of the spinal canal carry the feeling of pain from the head, neck, arms, chest and abdomen. Below this level the pain is located either in the lower back or in the legs. There are about ten of these nerves on each side. When so many nerves can be affected in such a relatively small area, is it any wonder that backache presents such an enormous

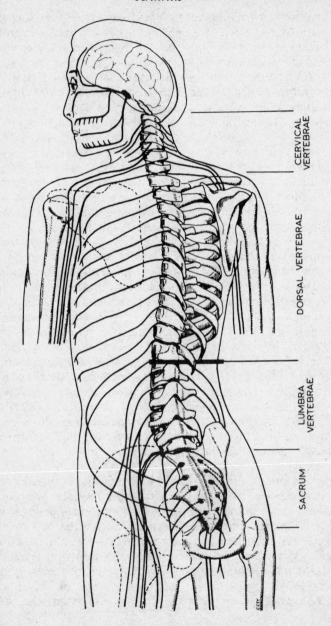

CERVICAL VERTEBRAE

DORSAL VERTEBRAE

LUMBRA VERTEBRAE

SACRUM

problem? If you think of the eight sets of nerves in the small area of the neck, you can see perhaps why 'migraine' presents so many variations, just as backache does. Perhaps we might call backache 'low-back migraine', not at all a bad description if you talk to some of the sufferers.

Here is one of my very first cases: A woman consulted me about pains in her back. She described these pains, how they woke her up night after night and had her pacing the room, how she had been to hospital, been examined and X-rayed and no diagnosis had been made (there was no evidence of arthritis on the X-ray). She was designated a neurotic. Tears were streaming down her face; unhappiness was written all over her. The demoralizing effect it was having on her, her husband and the children was just as important as the pain she suffered.

I felt pretty helpless but sent her home and went over to examine her thoroughly. Examination revealed nothing but some tender areas in the lumbar muscles of her back. Surely this was some kind of rheumatism, I thought, but I had had very little teaching on rheumatism and knew very little about it. She told me that big doses of aspirin gave her some relief, but she was unable to tolerate them. Reference to medical textbooks was fruitless, since there was no description of this type of pain and illness and obviously no suggestions for its diagnosis. Fortunately, at that time I read an article on the treatment of rheumatism by Dr Warren Crowe, who ran the Charterhouse Rheumatism Clinic in London, and decided to try a course of injections of his vaccine for this patient. She got very much better. I was not prepared to commit myself as to whether the vaccine treatment was effective, whether it coincided with a natural remission of the illness or whether a sympathetic doctor had relieved the tensions in the patient and the family by exorcism of the term 'neurotic'! Nevertheless, the outcome was highly satisfactory, for both the patient and myself. She was better, and I felt something had been done to help her. Again, I was tremendously impressed by the effect that the improvement had on the patient, her husband and her children.

As so many of my readers will know, this backache is

very common. You may not suffer as much as this poor woman because there is now such a variety of drugs to hide the pain or to dampen your sensitivity if the doctors think there is a 'neurotic' element. In retrospect it is quite obvious that this patient had a natural remission of her rheumatic condition which coincided with my treatment! Everybody knows how common backache is in the community. There is a Back Pain Association whose representatives appear on television at frequent intervals but do not offer much hope. The medical profession talk about back pain as if it were a diagnosis. Quite recently they had a symposium in Manchester entitled "What's New in Back Pain?". A report by Dr Colin Tudge in *World Medicine,* May 1978, indicated no real progress, but I liked his quotation from one of the speakers: "We don't really know what we're doing." Their main preoccupation is with the disc problem, which they do not seem to be able to solve.

Let me now give you three examples of such cases:

DISC? (1)
Mr P. C. aged 37

4th January 1967. He complained of chronic pain left base of spine for ten years, which had spread down to left ankle; his leg was stiff every morning when rising, eased later and stiffened after sitting. He was treated in hospital for a slipped disc: plaster jacket, belt, traction. No relief at all. He was never free from pain, tried an osteopath on and off for four years, but with no improvement. He had a history of pain in the right of his neck twenty years ago and occasional sore throats.

I gave him the usual injections into the rheumatic patches, which produced immediate improvement. His response was excellent, and within three weeks he was completely free of all symptoms. There were further attacks at increasing intervals which responded to treatment very quickly.

This patient's history started with neck pain and sore throat in 1947. Note the recurrence of pain and stiffness and the immediate response to treatment. After ten years of misery he now knows that any attack he gets will be aborted in a very short time. This is a case where a detailed history indicates the rheumatic nature of the condition and demonstrates how it can be mistaken for a slipped disc. The excellent and lasting results of treatment were due to the localized nature of the rheumatism, indicating a good resistance. The only drug he takes is an anti-histamine.

DISC? (2)
Mr V. P. aged 43
He had his first attack of lumbago in 1963, which cleared up after a while under the care of his GP, then a second attack two years later which did not get better. He was treated for slipped disc with rest, traction and plaster jacket, both as an in-patient and, later, as an out-patient for eight months, with no improvement at all.

I injected the rheumatic patches, with immediate relief of symptoms. After three treatments he was completely free from pain. He sustained slight recurrences which always responded to one or two local injections and so never had to miss his work. In 1968, and again in 1970, he had a generalized attack which responded well to a few days' rest and aspirin. He has remained absolutely free from all back pain since. The localized nature of the disease with only two generalized attacks at two-year intervals explains why his response was so good.

DISC? (3)
Mr J. B. aged 48
29th November 1971. He had had chronic lumbar backache for twenty years; it was worse on left side and had spread down to ankle. He sustained frequent acute attacks in his back, when he was unable to work, and was always stiff in the morning when getting out of bed; he felt constantly tired. His longest period free from actual pain was three to four days. He could not do odd jobs at home because of his back and tiredness and could take no part in any sport. He was awaiting admission to hospital for operation on his spine.

Treatment consisted of an injection into the rheumatic patch in the back, which gave immediate improvement in the left leg and back. Treatment continued three times weekly for two weeks and then at longer intervals. Within one month he was totally free from pain and stiffness. He could do anything and was happily redecorating his home after work. I saw him at six-monthly intervals for influenza vaccine. February 1973: he suffered pain in the back and left leg down to the ankle after moving furniture. The treatment was repeated. It cleared up completely in three to four weeks, and he has been perfectly well since.

If the original diagnosis of disc trouble had been accepted, the relapse after moving furniture would certainly be attributed to a recurrence of the 'disc' trouble. Careful questioning elicited the story that the pain was not of sudden onset whilst moving the furniture but only associated with it in his mind. This is an extremely important point in diagnosis. You must distinguish between pain which actually starts quite suddenly and stops the patient from doing something he was about to attempt. This is almost certainly an acute rheumatic incident. On the other hand, pain which is brought on when actually bending or lifting is more likely to be associated with a disc lesion. If this kind of analysis had been made of this patient's symptoms, twenty years of inactivity and misery could have been avoided, to say nothing of an operation which he has escaped.

This is another example of rheumatic pain in the lumbar and sacral areas being confused with disc lesions. When Orthopaedic Departments have learned to differentiate lumbo-sacral rheumatic patches from disc lesions, they will cut down their traction, plaster jackets and surgical belts by a considerable number, quite apart from saving the patients a good deal of misery and wasted time.

These three examples are cases wrongly diagnosed and treated as slipped disc in different hospitals. There are far more cases of backache which they cannot 'diagnose' because the symptoms do not fit any of their preconceived ideas. Many of these backaches are due to rheumatic patches. They can be readily located and many of them successfully treated. Because they are not recognized, investigation into the cause of the pain has attained ludicrous proportions. X-ray techniques can now detect fine hairline cracks in the vertebrae which it is thought might be the cause of the pain. Have these people never seen gross fractures of vertebra which can be found on routine X-rays of the back and which are not giving rise to pain? Why all this preoccupation with faulty posture, strain and X-ray pictures? These are all the results of a disease-process which starts with the rheumatic patches. Inflammation of these patches is the cause of the pain. Everything else is a logical progression and not the cause of the symptoms.

I include Group C cases in this chapter because they are very small in number and present a problem which can be resolved only by a doctor who can evaluate the knowledge of the known disease with the symptoms of the patient. This was my very first case in this category—about the same time as the first woman with backache. I was able to help this patient only because I had been studying osteopathy, a subject I shall discuss later on.

GROUP C
DISEASES WHERE TREATMENT OF THE DIAGNOSED DISEASE DID NOT IMPROVE THE SYMPTOMS

I was asked to visit a man aged forty-eight who was bed-ridden with a bad heart. He was suffering a good deal of pain over his heart, and no one had been able to help him; it was merely put down to the heart condition. After a consideration of his history and a full clinical examination, which revealed an enlarged heart with valvular disease, I concluded that the pains from which he was suffering could not be attributed to a heart that was being rested completely, as was his.

In this case, after 'thoroughly' examining the man, according to hospital teaching, I turned him over in the bed, this time to examine his back. Imagine my interest in finding a marked kyphosis of the spine (a sort of hunchback with arthritis of the spinal bones). I still remember the impression it made on me at that time, it was so vivid, so illuminating.

This man's pain had nothing at all to do with his heart. He

had neuralgia of the nerves in the chest wall over the heart, caused by irritation of the nerve in the region of the kyphosis. By manipulating his spine, the pain was very much relieved. A continuation of this treatment a few times, over the course of about two or three weeks, and the man was able to get about with no pain at all. A very interesting aspect of his illness was that the valvular disease of the heart was due to rheumatic fever, whilst the arthritis in his spine was also a rheumatic condition. What a logical explanation for two 'different' diseases in the same person!

It is admitted that there are at least 3 million arthritics in this country alone. This diagnosis is accepted only when X-ray evidence is produced.

After reading these chapters, is there any doubt that there must be an equal, or even larger, number who have the same disease before X-ray changes can possibly take place? Add to these all those people with 'allied diseases', some of whom are undoubtedly to be found in cardiac, orthopaedic and psychiatric departments, and you have a daunting picture of the enormous mass of ill-health which affects this nation.

Without doing any more than scrapping the wasteful expenditure on outmoded treatment of arthritis, such as physiotherapy and massive amounts of drugs, and replacing it by my methods, enough money and manpower would be saved to provide as many kidney machines as are needed, with all the necessary services. In addition, waiting-lists for 'non-urgent' operations would be decimated. What a world of misery and anxiety the expression 'non-urgent' hides! People who need hip operations— because of the failure of rheumatological treatment—can be made reasonably pain-free, mobile and independent; is that not urgent enough? Operations for hernias, which affect the activity of so many—are they not urgent? As I suggested earlier in the book, what doctors may consider are not 'major' or even 'urgent' diseases very often do not correspond with the viewpoint of the patients. I believe there is too wide a gap between the patients and the profession due to that lack of dialogue which I am trying to bridge.

8

Differences Among Doctors

There was a time when lawsuits for damages in cases of injury or illness made the headlines in the newspapers, because there were conflicting views by medical witnesses on the same case. Such situations are now commonplace but rarely heard about. The insurance companies have found it cheaper to settle cases at a reasonable level rather than face heavy legal costs due to these conflicting views. Furthermore, the expert witness retained by the insurance company is a formidable obstacle which the injured party's advisers are often unable to challenge.

Lay people find it difficult to understand why doctors can disagree about what should be hard facts in any given medical case. The reason is, however, easily explained when you realize, from what I have already said, that there is so much of which they are not aware.

How widespread is this lack of knowledge can be illustrated in the following case which involves a patient, a hospital, a physician, an orthopaedic surgeon, a rheumatologist and myself. For me it was a critical test as to whether my theories and practice of the rheumatic disease would stand up to the most searching analysis which only time can present.

In June 1967, following a motor accident, Mr L. C. E.,
aged twenty-three was admitted to hospital with the
following injuries: severe concussion lasting about thirty-
six hours; damage to his jaws, with loss of some teeth;
fracture of the knuckle joint in the right index finger;
fracture of the pelvis and a flake of bone in the right hip
joint. After discharge as an in-patient, he attended the
physiotherapy department for heat, exercise and massage
three times a week and was given various drugs for the
pain. After some months of this treatment he asked his
solicitor if he could recommend him to a specialist because
he was not improving and used to come away from his
treatment literally crying with pain. His solicitor was a
patient and a friend of mine and knew a good deal about my
work. He asked me if I could see him and give an opinion as
to what I thought should be done, either by me or by
referring him elsewhere.

I first saw the young man on 28th February 1968. His
complaints were as follows:

1. Constant ache in the neck with severe headaches lasting
   up to three days. They sometimes improved after a nose-
   bleed.
2. Constant pain in the back so that he could not sit
   normally, always adjusting his position to avoid
   pressure.
3. Pain over right hip, variable.
4. Weakness of the right index finger, which made writing
   very difficult.
5. Very bad-tempered, even quarrelling with his brother,
   which he had never done previously. He knew he was
   being very difficult in the office; all this was quite foreign
   to him.
6. He continued to have dreadful nightmares.

The flake of bone in the hip joint and the fracture of the
pelvis were no longer visible. X-ray of his neck and back
showed no signs of injury or disease. After a thorough
examination, I reported to his solicitor that the pain and
weakness of the finger, the neck pain and headaches, and
the pain in the back, were all due to the same cause. A
widespread attack of rheumatism which had affected all

these areas was due, undoubtedly, to the shock of the accident and damage to the soft tissues. There were rheumatic patches everywhere. That was why the massage and exercises were making him worse. I said further that he would need at least three years to recover completely, if at all, and that the present treatment must be stopped. Imagine massage and exercises being given to inflamed areas! It was no wonder that he was reduced to tears. I predicted that, unless the disease could be controlled, he would develop arthritis, which is accepted by the profession only on X-ray evidence.

Within a week or two, a physician, representing the insurance company against whom there was a claim for the accident, requested a joint consultation with me, after seeing my report. I knew the physician quite well—I had met him on other cases. After he had examined the patient, in my presence, we sent him away and had a little chat. The physician had no doubt at all that the lad was malingering; he was only after compensation. As he said, there was now no X-ray evidence of damage or arthritis—everything was healed. I tried to explain my views, but I am afraid he could not be bothered to listen.

I continued to treat this patient, who was showing some definite signs of getting better. He never failed to report any improvement he noticed. The tranquillizers were discarded and also some of the pain-relievers.

A few weeks later a second consultation took place, this time with an orthopaedic surgeon representing the insurance company. Do I need to tell you? Further X-rays were taken: no disease was shown, so there was nothing wrong with the patient. The same opinion expressed: "He is malingering; he is only after compensation." I knew the surgeon very well and had great respect for his surgical skill, so much so that I had sent several cases to him for treatment. I pointed out to him that he had examined the patient only from the point of view of the bones and that it was the ligament and connective tissue which were causing the symptoms. I further pointed out that the patient had improved under my care and that he must know very well that I was not the sort of person to take fees for work unless I was sure I was doing the right thing. It was of no use: he still persisted in his belief that the patient was malingering. In September 1971, I had a second consultation with the same surgeon. The same view of malingering was expressed. The patient was very much better but still had some headaches and backache.

Following this consultation the insurance company offered some puny compensation and was not prepared to pay my medical fees. Because the patient could not afford to pay my fees, he thanked me for all I had done and said he would try to carry on as best he could. Neither he nor his solicitor had any doubts about my judgement, and they accepted my advice not to settle but to go to court.

The case was due to be heard in the High Court in September 1974.

Whilst preparing the medical evidence, I told the solicitor that, although I knew I was right, my evidence ought to be backed up by a rheumatologist of some standing. After all, I was not attached to a hospital and did not possess a specialist degree, and the eminent surgeon and the physician, who believed the patient to be a malingerer, might impress the judge more than I could hope to do. This was agreed, and I invited such a rheumatologist to examine the patient and see if we agreed about his condition. After a good deal of discussion, he agreed there was some evidence of rheumatism but was rather insistent that there was a psychological factor involved—should we not, perhaps, have a psychiatrist? I said I would prefer not to complicate the problem, because the psychiatric part was, in my view, due to all the anxiety caused by the prolonged proceedings—we were now in the sixth year. So it was agreed that his evidence would be restricted to the fact that there was some evidence of rheumatism.

A few days before the hearing, the orthopaedic surgeon decided to have a final set of X-rays of the patient. To his credit, he phoned me to say that I could see the X-rays, as there was, for the first time, evidence of very early arthritis, in the neck bones—exactly what I had predicted six years before. Nevertheless, he said it was only slight and still did not think it was really significant, or at least that is what he said to me on the Friday before the case.

The following Tuesday, fifteen minutes before the case was to be heard, the insurance company agreed to a very substantial settlement of the case, which certainly pleased the patient and counsel. The sad part of the case was that the solicitor, who had shown so much faith in my opinion, died some time before it was settled.

The point of telling this case in detail is to show that:

1. A physician did not believe this man because he did not understand the nature of rheumatism.
2. For the same reason I was unable, even in three long interviews, to convince the orthopaedic surgeon of the true nature of the disease.
3. Even the rheumatologist found it difficult entirely to accept what I said, and he wanted an escape in psychiatry in case things went wrong at the trial. This was, of course, before we had the final X-rays.

The failure of rheumatologists to recognize or understand the early manifestations of these diseases can be further illustrated by two more cases.

The first case concerns a young girl (at school) who developed pains in the back when playing tennis. She was a very good player and extremely keen. After an examination I explained to the girl, Angela, and her mother, that she had rheumatism affecting the ligament and connective tissue of the spine. It was not a very active condition, but exercise was aggravating it. Although Angela was very upset, on my advice she gave up tennis and restricted the amount of physical exercise she did at school if and when her back troubled her. With this regime, she needed very little treatment and went through school collecting several certificates on the way.

At sixteen she made up her mind that she wanted to be a nurse, and nothing was going to stop her. She was that lovely, sweet type of girl on whom the nursing profession depends, a vocational girl to whom money and heavy work meant very little. Because of her rheumatism, her mother was very worried as to what the arduous work would do to her back. She had already told Angela of her concern. We had a long discussion, and I came to the conclusion that

Angela would never forgive either her parents or me if we vetoed her entry to nursing. She would never believe that she could not do it. Therefore, I advised that she be allowed to try, and we could review the situation in the light of experience. She was accepted as a trainee in a famous teaching hospital.

All went well for a while, but as soon as she had to do heavy work, lifting patients etc, her back began to give trouble. She came to see me in tears, not so much because of the pain but because she did not want to give up nursing. I treated her and wrote a note to the Medical Registrar at the hospital, suggesting that she be excused heavy work. She was accordingly referred to the Head of the Rheumatology Department. X-rays and blood-tests were carried out. She was examined by the consultant and pronounced free from all rheumatic taint! Naturally, her mother came to see me; who was she to believe? As she put it, "You have been telling me for years that Angela has rheumatism, and now a specialist at this teaching hospital says absolutely no, she should be able to do all her duties." I said what a pity it was that Angela did not ask what was the cause of her pains, if not rheumatism. But what nurse, and in this case a student nurse, would have the temerity to question a consultant!

However, both mother and daughter were content to trust me. We received marvellous co-operation from the Sister Tutor at the hospital—unofficially, of course. Angela was able to avoid the heavy work most of the time. She came for treatment when the rheumatic patches flared up, eventually qualified as a nurse and then as a sister.

Recall my first case of backache, in Darwen: no X-ray evidence of arthritis—the woman was neurotic. Over thirty years later, the same attitude to rheumatism persisted. Is it any wonder that there is no progress!

The second case concerns a sister at another teaching hospital. The story is recorded here in her own words.

In July 1974 I went to an orthopaedic surgeon for pain, stiffness and swelling of the index and middle fingers of the left hand. He diagnosed trigger finger, and for two weeks I had hot wax baths and ultrasonic treatment, with no improvement. The hand was operated on—afterwards the surgeon told me it was not trigger finger, that all appeared normal, apart from swelling of the tendons, and that he really did not know what was wrong. The pain and stiffness persisted. I continued to see the surgeon, who then gave me some Butozolidine for the swelling—but again, no improvement. Blood-tests and X-rays were done. Everything was negative.

After three months the surgeon thought perhaps I had an 'atypical rheumatoid' and referred me to a consultant rheumatologist at a major London teaching hospital. Once more all the blood-tests and X-rays were taken and found to be negative. I was started on Indocid, which I took for 1½ years with no effect. In November 1974 the thumb joint on the right hand became affected, and by January 1975 the thumb on the left hand became similarly affected, i.e. pain, stiffness, swelling and terrific throbbing. More X-rays and blood-tests were taken, and again all were normal. I was tried on other drugs, one of which brought me out in a rash after twenty-four hours and had to be stopped. I was then tried on another drug, which was ineffective, and was also given one injection of cortisone into the worst-affected joint—the left index finger. Things continued along in this way for seven to eight months, with my hands becoming more swollen, painful and stiff. The Indocid was increased to 125 mgs each night. Blood-tests and X-rays were repeated at six-monthly intervals, and all were still negative. It was suggested at this point that perhaps I was allergic to the contraceptive pill. Things got no better, and I was becoming more and more worried.

In October 1975 I requested another opinion and was duly referred to another senior rheumatologist at another major London teaching hospital. The usual examinations, blood-tests and X-rays were carried out. All were negative. I was started on various other drugs, including one which worked havoc with my mental condition, and I finally ended up taking Brufen 2 Tabs tds.

By March 1976 definite bone-changes were noticed on X-ray. By this time my hands were causing me an enormous amount of pain—the simplest things were very difficult to do, i.e. opening doors, fitting keys in locks, picking up books from a table, answering the telephone. The weight of bedclothes I could not bear, and getting washed and dressed was an ordeal. The cleaning of my teeth had to be postponed to lunchtime as I just could not use the tooth-brush first thing in the morning. Life was really miserable—my work suffered, as I could not do anything of a practical nature to look after my patients. I was desperately tired all the time—all my spare time was spent in bed trying to gain enough energy to go on duty. I looked very pale and drawn—all my friends were convinced I had anaemia. But my Hb reports came back consistently good, 11–13 grms.

In view of the continuing failure of treatment offered me, a rheumatologist suggested a choice of three other treat-ments: anti-malarial drugs, penicillamine or gold injections. I was terrified out of my life, rejected all three and never went back to that rheumatologist again. As a nurse I had seen enough of that kind of treatment, particularly gold, to make me very reluctant even to try them.

I really did not know what to do next. I had been to two of the best-known and most respected rheumatologists in London, and all I could honestly say was that I was very much worse than when I started. My hands would settle down for a week or two and then flare up worse than ever. Life seemed very bleak. I was thirty-five. I am a nurse and depend on my hands for my livelihood.

One day in May 1976 a friend gave me a book on arthritis by a Dr William W. Fox. I was a bit sceptical. Why was he not attached to a big London teaching hospital? Why were his methods not used more widely? However, after a particu-larly nasty bout of pain I swallowed my scepticism one day and rang him. He agreed to see me. That was a year ago. Since then I have improved enormously. The damaged joints, i.e. damaged before I got to him, are almost *unrecog-nizable*, and the rest of my hands look perfect. I can now do most of the things I could not do before. Delicate move-ments and actions are no longer torture. His treatment has worked wonderfully for me. It has been painful, but it *works*. Dr Fox explains your disease to you. He is completely honest. He is sympathetic and understanding and likes all his patients to have a full explanation and understanding of his treatment.

An important part of his treatment involves rest when a disease is active. Some six months ago I started to run a temperature of 37·3–37·6 every day. I felt absolutely listless, just as I did before; pains developed in my arms and legs.

He explained that this was a period when the disease was trying to reassert itself. Until my natural resistance to the disease-process developed, with whatever help he could give me, rest was imperative. He requested three months' leave of absence from my GP, who, although sympathetic, suggested I see yet another rheumatologist. I had to agree, as otherwise she would not give me the certificate.

I was examined by yet another consultant rheumatologist in another major teaching hospital, who said, at the end of his examination, that I might have had rheumatoid but that it was now gone. My temperature was, he said, "of no consequence—lots of people had temperatures—we don't worry about them," and finally he recommended that I see a psychiatrist as I was suffering from depression. (In fairness to him, I must say that I was depressed. I had some problems in my personal life that were worrying me, and I did agree to see a psychiatrist. Dr Fox was fully aware of my personal problems. He pointed out that they had been with me a long time and had not stopped me getting better up until this relapse.) What struck me most of all was the consultant's utter inability to accept that I had rheumatoid because the symptoms displayed were not what he was used to seeing in his patients. I was given the impression that I was malingering. The facts, that for three months I had had a low-grade temperature and was utterly devoid of energy, mattered not at all. Because I was not disfigured and only in pain meant that I was not suffering from rheumatoid arthritis. Yet all those who know me and work with me agree that my improvement over the last year has been nothing short of dramatic. Some of the doctors with whom I work used to say to me, "Never mind, it will burn itself out after leaving you with disfigured joints." Well, some of them still say, "It's burned itself out" but they are a bit mystified as to what happened to the disfigured joints!

Needless to say, I did not get leave of absence and so struggled on until I had a holiday period, when I was able to rest. The period of remission since the holiday seemed now to be slowly coming along. The temperature is at last subsiding; my hands have maintained their improvement, and many of the other pains in my neck and legs are settling down.

The story of my disease is exactly as Dr Fox describes in his book. The continuing deterioration of my condition until

I consulted him, together with the remarkable progress I have made (almost precisely as he predicted), has changed my outlook completely, even though I still have the same personal problems. I dread to think what my hands would have been like without Dr Fox's treatment. I believe it is possible for this dread to be turned into hope, real hope, if my message can get through to those who have the power and responsibility. Ah! Dear patients—hope not too much!

Because I am a qualified sister, Dr Fox has allowed me to meet quite a number of his patients. The story is ever the same—endless treatment with no improvement until he started his own treatment. Knowing how sceptical I was before consulting him, I realize the profession must have the same doubts as to his claims. May I say to them what Dr Fox said to me when I first consulted him: "What have you got to lose?"

You will recall how I described the manner in which the human body was divided into about twenty-five separate specialities for the purpose of studying and treating diseases. You will also remember how I indicated that, broadly speaking, the various specialists never really came together and that for almost all of them nothing existed but the diseases in which they specialized, so that if a patient did not have their particular disease, then that patient really did not exist for them. A patient who had exhausted the specialities which remotely resembled his or her symptoms was now left with nowhere to go.

The limited knowledge of the general practitioner, together with even more limited time and patience, means that the treatment would be back to the 'bad old days' of counteracting symptoms, but with the added danger of hiding the true symptoms with pain-killers and tranquillizers. These drugs can, and often do, produce undesirable side-effects which add to the patients' misery and serve further to confuse the whole clinical picture. There is now no hope of any doctor achieving a diagnosis in terms of known physical disease, so all that is left is psychiatry.

The psychiatrists are now taking on all those cases where no *known* physical disease exists. This is not the same as saying that there is *no* physical disease. If what I have told you in this book has any truth at all, it means that countless

numbers of people are likely to be referred to the psychiatrists simply because their organic or physical disease has
not been recognized. So a patient starts with the psychiatrist on the positive assumption that there is no physical
disease causing the depression, etc. There is no clear defini-
tion of what represents a normal human mind—how can
there be when we are all so different? I suppose each
psychiatrist will consider that normality is a state of mind
which has a close resemblance to his or her own. If you were
to think about yourself and reflect on the different moods
which have affected you over, say, the last month, how
often would you be able to say, "Oh! I didn't realize I could
be like that." Think how you reacted to different people and
differing situations, how some people bring out the best in
you and others the worst, whatever that may be. How
many doctors stop to think that the worried patient in the
consulting-room is really not the same person who lives at
home with his family or friends? Changes in mood and
personality depend in varying degrees on environmental
factors, at home, at school or at work. Judging from my
experience in talking with patients, the very idea of having
to consult a doctor often causes more violent emotional
changes in them than environmental factors. Fear of what
might be and anxiety as to the future are just two emotions
which do not normally affect you, but at this stage they do,
and so the doctor is not seeing you as you really are. If,
added to these adverse circumstances, you also have a pain
or ache, or depression which 'does not exist' because it
cannot be diagnosed, what possible chance can there be of a
psychiatrist even understanding you?

Here is an example of psychiatric diagnostic error that I
encountered some years ago.

Alice was a young married woman who had been a
patient of mine since the age of sixteen and whom I saw
only rarely because she was fit and well. Her husband
turned out to have some mental disorder for which he was
regularly treated at a well-known hospital. He certainly
caused her a great deal of mental strain, but she coped
exceedingly well without any drugs. She was holding down
a very responsible job. Then, in the summer of that year she

became very ill and depressed whilst staying with her parents in Birmingham and was under the local doctor. She eventually returned to London and was soon referred by her GP to the same hospital as that which her husband attended. She was admitted and treated as a psychiatric case for something like three months.

When I returned from holiday, her parents contacted me and begged me to see her. I agreed, of course, and when she arrived at my consulting-room, I could hardly believe it was the same girl I had known for so many years. She was heavily drugged and showed practically no reaction; her face was like a mask, and she showed no emotion whatever. A detailed history showed that she must have had a severe virus infection in Birmingham, like a severe influenza. You recall my own story when in the 1930s there was an influenza epidemic which killed thousands because of its severity, and there was also a considerable number of suicides and attempted suicides by patients who were greatly depressed by the illness. So why be surprised if it happens today?

I treated the patient by telling her what I believed to be the truth. I gave her a course of vitamins and stopped all the drugs. Within three to four weeks she was back at work. She has never been ill since, except for a few twinges of rheumatism. She has an even more responsible job and copes with all her domestic problems.

It seems to me that psychiatrists are attempting to explain in psychological terms an illness which may have a physical basis of which they are unaware, with symptoms which are aggravated by the patient's anxiety and confusion. The anxiety and confusion have been generated by the failure of the GP and specialist to understand the true nature of the illness.

Remember the surgeon who could find no diagnosis for many cases of abdominal pain? He, at least, was concerned about the problem, but no doubt some of his patients ended up in the psychiatric department. Around that same time a child-specialist at Ancoats Hospital, near Manchester, wrote an article which also appeared in the *Lancet*. He reported the number of children referred to him with vague pains in an arm or leg for which he could find no explanation. He was worried for the same reason as the surgeon. It is highly unsatisfactory to a thinking person not to be able to understand those symptoms. Neither of these writers thought to designate the patients as neurotic or psychiatric. Perhaps their minds were more in tune with mine, believing that people do not invent symptoms—they have them—even children have them!

More recently, a child-specialist, Professor John Apley of Bristol who sadly has since died had been reported as calling children coming under his care "little bellyachers". Their symptoms varied between vague pains in the arm or leg like growing-pains, stomach pains, headache and even migraine. Apparently only one in twenty of the stomach cases produced evidence of organic disease. His conclusion was that in all the other cases the pain originated in the child's mind, which was linked to stress and worries in the family and possibly to some hereditary factor. I am quite sure that in the present state of medical knowledge Dr Apley was fully justified in assuming that these children have no known physical basis for their complaints. In that context his conclusions seem very reasonable. But I hope it would not seem libellous for me to suggest that it is just possible that a re-examination of these patients, based on the new knowledge of the rheumatic patch, might reveal such a physical condition in some of the cases.

I have been a doctor in active practice for nearly fifty years. I cannot count the number of children I have looked after. Never have I seen a child in pain for which I could not find a physical cause. If you are talking about stress, strain and anxiety, I spent seven years in Darwen in the 1930s where unemployment was 42 per cent and where the Welfare State did not exist. I saw hundreds of children with constant coughs, colds, bronchitis and aching legs and arms. The reason they were ill was because they were literally starved of basic food and vitamins, warmth and clothing, which most certainly does not happen today. I have been in too many homes and attended too many children to believe that children decide to imagine they have a pain in a particular place. Why should one decide to have it in the arm, another a leg, a third in the stomach and a fourth in the head? Exaggeration of a pain I might accept from an unhappy or spoilt child, but pain there must be in the first place.

You, dear reader, can try a simple experiment. Try to convince yourself that you have a pain in any part of the body you choose. Try as hard as you can for as long as you can. You will never succeed in persuading your brain that you have a pain. How, then, do you suppose that a mere child could succeed in such self-deception? What desperate mental harm may be done to a child whose parents, teachers and doctors are all of the opinion possibly suggested by the doctor, that the pain, although real, is 'imaginary'.

There is hardly one case of arthritis of any kind that does not recall growing-pains in childhood. It is the earliest sign of rheumatism in children. That pain could just as easily be in arm, head or stomach.

Try to imagine yourself back in childhood, with a pain in your head, and constantly being told there is no cause for it except in your mind. What an awful effect this could have on your mind and personality. I do not think we should worry overmuch about stresses and strains in the home. Children are conditioned to them and probably do not know that they are abnormal. How does a child of five or six compare his experiences with other children? The answer is that he does not; his environment is the only one he knows. Except in the very worst homes, of which there cannot be too many, mothers have a natural instinct of love and protection for their offspring, just like the animals in the wild. (Maybe the animals are lucky not to have a free medical service!)

In the adult world, I wonder how many of you saw, three years ago on the television, a doctor from the Midlands discussing the problem of backache in car-workers. Backache is a common problem there—where is it not? As I recall, this is the gist of what he said. They were all investigated and X-rayed. If the pictures showed evidence of arthritis, then they were given appropriate treatment—whatever that might be. If, however, there was no X-ray evidence of arthritis, then the accent on treatment would be on the 'nervous' side. He also talked about job-boredom as a possible cause! Forgive me this question: Is it like "The Charge of the Back Brigade—Forward the 'Valium' 600"? Believe me, this is no exaggeration. Practically every new patient I have seen in the last ten years has been taking Valium or similar drugs, in addition to pain-killers.

Three cases: Alice, who had been a psychiatric patient; Mr L. C. E., who went through the courts, and Susan F., who had 'strange' tummy pains, especially at school, have all been resolved by a realization of what was really wrong with them, undiagnosed rheumatic conditions. There have, of course, been many more cases through my hands, not quite as serious but extremely important to the individuals concerned.

In contrast to these three cases, I should like to tell you about a lady who consulted me about her back pains some years ago.

She came 70 miles to see me. After hearing the history and doing an examination, I came to the conclusion that her rheumatism was really quite mild and could hardly account for her depression. I explained to her that I did not think her condition merited a course of treatment which meant this long journey, perhaps twice weekly. I suggested in the kindliest way that perhaps there was some other cause for the depression, and would she like to discuss this possibility. There was a sudden burst of tears, and then came the real truth. Her husband was an alcoholic and knocked her about when he was drunk. The backache was the excuse she used for her depression to her friends, one of whom had recommended her to come and see me. We discussed the matter, and I gave her an appointment only on condition that her husband had been told and that he would come along with her. She later phoned to confirm the arrangement. When she arrived the following week, it was difficult to believe she was the same woman. She looked younger, happier and really quite bright. Her husband was quiet and very gentlemanly. He listened to all I had to say and agreed to give up drink. At her next appointment I asked her how her husband had reacted to my lecture. She replied, "Do

you really want me to tell you?'' I answered in the affirma-
tive, and this is what he said, ''I would like to punch that
bloody doctor on the nose for being right!'' Things went
excellently after that and her husband sent me some senior
members of his staff for treatment! I wish I could say that it
was 'happy ever after'. Alas, the drink problem returned,
and the inevitable divorce duly took place.

Now you can see two sides of the psychiatric problem,
the one caused by the failure of the doctors to diagnose a
physical condition, and the other where domestic and
personal problems do affect what can be quite a minor
illness.

There is even a third side to this 'eternal problem'. . .

An old patient of mine telephoned to ask if I could recommend a good psychiatrist. He explained that his married
sister had become a great problem and burden to her family
and was threatening suicide. Her GP referred her to
hospital, but, as is not unusual in this era, people are scared
of these last-ditch diagnoses and treatments. He understood my professional attitude not to interfere with other
doctors' services, and it was left at that. A week or so later,
he rang again. His sister suffered a lot from arthritis, and
perhaps I would see her about this, as she was in a lot of
pain—it might have some bearing on her depression. I
agreed to see her.

A detailed history revealed that five years earlier she had
told her doctor that she had a swelling of her left ankle.
From then on until now she had been taking 'water pills'
and Slow K, every single day. The swelling had never been
very much, and there was little visible when I saw her. She
had rheumatic patches in her leg, and I had no doubt that
the original swelling in her ankle was a rheumatic condition. I treated her with local injections, which improved
the leg. I advised the complete cessation of the 'water pills'
and Slow K, and within one week all her psychiatric
troubles were over.

So not only do some doctors cause psychiatric problems
by not understanding their patients' symptoms, but they
actually create them by giving drugs for which there is no
need and which affect the psyche. Evidence is daily

accumulating of the adverse effects of drugs. They have been given a medical designation, 'atrogenic disease'. Recently, a physician in one hospital has been so perplexed at the strange multiplicity of symptoms in his patients that he clears the ground, so to speak, by taking them off all drugs in order to discover what their real symptoms are.

The link in all these cases is the rheumatic story I have tried to describe in this book. It is manifestly impossible to have contrived all this evidence, substantiated in so many different cases. Therefore, I believe that none of your suffering will prove to be necessary when all these various specialists realize that there are sound, orthodox, clinical facts of which they were not aware but which they can verify.

9

The National Health Service

As early as 1931 I started the idea of co-operation between the general practitioners in Darwen, and when I came to London in 1937, I spoke about it to a British Medical Association meeting of the St Pancras Division. I told them how successful the experiment had been in Darwen and suggested that we might try it here. What a reception I got! Almost every doctor who spoke had the 'dog in the manger' attitude: most of the discussion centred on how much a doctor would be paid for doing a visit for another doctor. I explained that in Darwen the question of fees was dismissed because we all realized that over a long period what we did for each other would balance out. The money was not important; it was the freedom from responsibility for the odd day or two which was so vital to the well-being of the doctor. I knew it was impossible to work six full days a week plus night calls and always some visits on the Sunday without its having a bad affect on one's health and concentration. The patients were bound to suffer a diminution of the standard of service from a tired doctor. I also told them of the bonus of being able to discuss the cases we had seen: that two heads were better than one was proved sometimes to be a good idea. It was of no avail. The doctors in London turned it down. Most of them did not know each other; they lived and practised in isolation, except for the occasional professional meetings of the local BMA groups, which were very infrequent and very sparsely attended. It was obvious that many doctors were not making a very good living and preferred to remain permanently on call for their patients.

I remember being told by a newspaper reporter that in some areas, especially the East End, a patient in need of urgent treatment would phone two or three doctors, and the first one to arrive got the job! There was also the celebrated story of the doctor who had a notice in his waiting-room which read "Consultation 1/6 (one shilling and six-pence)—with stethoscope 2/- (two shillings)." I think he overvalued his stethoscope service! In those days you could get a very prompt service, which is quite the opposite from today, as you all know. "Ah! But you are getting a much better service today," will be the retort. Before I discuss this statement, I think you should know a little of my own activities in medical politics.

During the war I lived and worked in London. When I was not out on emergency duty during air-raids, I sat with my wife in the sand-bag-reinforced consulting-room at home. We had sent our two children, aged seven and five, to Canada. The Canadians were marvellous to them, but we both suffered great deprivation. I turned first to the Bible and then to philosophy, both of which I read avidly during the long, dimly lit hours of the air-raids. I was seeking for some explanation for man's inhumanity to man, an answer to the riddle of eternal sin. I did not find it, but I did learn a great deal which sustained me through those dreadful days and which spurred me on to work for a National Health Service. In retrospect, I realize that I was a certain candidate for this idea.

The present generation cannot possibly understand the change which the war and Churchill wrought on the people of this country. Because of our common danger, people really cared far more for each other than ever seemed possible in that supposedly class-ridden society. Unfortunately, we are back with those prejudices now, but the accent is on different classes of privilege and power—that, however, is another story. The concern for others at that time was so widespread that Lord Beveridge, a great Liberal leader in his time, was commissioned to produce his famous Beveridge Report, on which the pattern of the New Britain was to be based. The twin pillars of his recommendations were full employment and a comprehensive National Health Service. Not being a politician, but caring about people, I devoted much of my 'leisure' to promoting the need for a National Health Service. The BMA membership was substantially against it and bitterly opposed to a salaried service. The Socialist Medical Society was all for the National Health Service, and therefore I became a member. I was appointed Chairman of its Health Centre Committee.

The Health Centre was to be a place where doctors had full ancillary staff and would not be involved with all the clerical problems which beset the ordinary GP, thus giving them much more time to devote to each patient. Many minor investigations could be done there instead of overloading the hospitals, and which would make work more interesting for the doctors. The latter would also have a meeting-place where they could discuss problems of diagnosis, treatment and administration. Best of all, there would be accommodation where doctors could give popular lectures on simple anatomy, health and disease. That would teach them how to communicate with their patients in simple terms, and the patients would learn more about themselves and so communicate better with the doctors.

I was so keen on this concept that I joined forces with three other doctors, and we became candidates for the Council of the British Medical Association to represent London. Miracle of miracles! We were elected. Now I was at the heart of the BMA, I could, with my colleagues, persuade them of the wonder of the new Health Service. Well, we may have been at the heart of the BMA, but it was the minds we wanted, and that was what we could not get. I remember addressing a Delegate Conference of the BMA of over three hundred medical representatives from all over Great Britain, on the importance of accepting the principle of a National Health Service. I warned them that the people wanted it and that it would be brought in, whether they liked it or not. I said it would be much better for the doctors to participate and help to plan a service which would be in their interest. Unless their reasonable needs were satisfied, the service would suffer. So far, there had been only a few derisory noises from the audience, but when I said, "There is nothing wrong with a salary—providing it is adequate," they did not hear the last four words—the noise of disapproval and the stamping drowned them. 'Salaried service' was an anathema to them. When I left the platform, a reporter from the *Daily Mail* approached me. We had a chat and I remember his telling me that it was shocking to see so many grown men behaving like schoolboys—and they were all doctors who could not listen to a reasoned argument. It does not surprise me any more, and perhaps it will not surprise you by the time you have finished the book.

Let us return to the more enlightened members of the medical profession—the Council of the Socialist Medical Association. We were fast approaching the time when Aneuran Bevan, the Health Minister, was determined to bring in the National Health Service. He was a very clever and able man. He split the profession in half—the specialists were all in favour, because now they were to be paid much more than ever they had dreamed of. If they were in the old poor-law and non-teaching hospitals, their salary had been about £800 per annum, and now it was to be £2,000 plus. The hierarchy in the teaching hospitals were to get similar salaries for work they had done before for nothing. The lame ducks—the GPs—were to continue as before, with a capitation fee, but with no Health Centres. They were really more like sheep who had lost their shepherd. They were 'baa-ing' against a salaried service, whilst the specialists were willing and ready to grasp the shekels, even if it was called a salary.

I think I was the only 'lame duck' on the Council of the Socialist Medical Association. I asked them why they were accepting the National Health Service without any place for Health Centres. I reminded them that our official policy had stated quite clearly that Health Centres were the linchpin of the new Service; without these the service would never succeed. The various specialists on the Council all agreed that we should not embarrass the Minister by insisting on Health Centres. Well, their cake had been nicely baked, so it was difficult to stop them from taking their slice. Because I was convinced the service would never reach anything like the standard I had worked and hoped for and that it would even demean medical practice, I resolved not to join the scheme. I could be no part of an organization which did not fulfil the preconditions necessary for better medical practice. I also resigned from the Council of the Socialist Medical Association.

All my medical friends and associates told me I was a fool and that I would be unable to make a living outside the service. Perhaps I understood the problems and human nature better than they. A large number of my patients wanted to try the free service. I agreed that by all means they should try it. However, if, after trying it, they wished to return to me, they should not feel embarrassed in so doing. Not unexpectedly, in the first year my income dropped like a stone. After that the rising graph of success never left me. When people have freedom of choice, they know on what they would rather spend their money.

I do hope that my readers will appreciate the sense and sincerity of all I have said. My great desire was, and still is, to help people. Perhaps this report, which appeared in the *News Chronicle* on 16th October 1945, will tell you more about my work than I can—for I was the doctor. The paper had only four pages, and this article appeared on the leader page.

News Chronicle, Tuesday, 16th October 1945
A Day in the Life of a Doctor
Civilian doctors are overworked. Many at home are breaking down under the strain of looking after two thousand or more patients. But doctors in the Services have too little work; the RAF, with no battle casualties, still maintains a ratio of one doctor to 430 men. Many medical officers in the Forces are bored and dissatisfied. But what does the situation mean to the doctor at home? Louise Morgan here tells the story of one day in the life of one typical London physician.

He is a typical London GP, one of the civilian few who are throwing everything they have into the struggle to guard the country's health. With no help, save what his wife can spare from her household duties and their children, he runs one surgery in his Highgate home, another in Kentish Town and a consulting-room in the West End. His panel is over seven hundred but brings him in less than £400 a year. Private practice yields him £2,400, but a substantial amount of this goes into subsidizing his panel practice, because he likes to treat all his patients alike.

Yesterday he allowed me to share his working day in order to record it as a piece of social documentation. Before we started off in his car at 9 am, he had spent an hour giving diagnoses, directions for treatment and 'a spot of comfort and cheer' on the telephone. He lies down while telephoning, to conserve his strength for the day.

We went to Hampstead Garden Suburb, where in the same family a mother had asthma, a daughter rheumatism and another daughter an abscess in the back.

"Be my timekeeper, will you?" he asked, as we left them at 9.20. "I'll have to concentrate on driving to fit all my visits in."

At 9.28 we were with a pair of distraught parents in Hampstead who had had little sleep since the birth of their infant. "It's they, not the baby, who need treatment," the doctor commented. It was the longest visit of the day and consisted of a straight but sympathetic talk on infant-management and a demonstration of how to handle a baby.

While there, a message reached him about a minor accident on the other edge of Hampstead.

"How's the time?" he asked anxiously as we hurried to the car, his stethoscope trailing, his rather thin hair flying.

"Sorry, it's almost ten."

He gripped the wheel and glued his eyes on the road. "Must cut out two visits. Remind me to telephone about them, will you?" I stayed outside while he dealt with the accident. Moving on at 10.20, he planned aloud. "I really must see that Merchant Navy boy today. It's on the way to the surgery. Haven't seen him for three weeks, and he counts on me. Queer, he was passed A1 when he joined up three years ago."

In a bright little flat, we found the patient—at twenty-eight a shadow of a man from TB. He, his young wife and the baby of eighteen months greeted the doctor as if he were Father Christmas.

We reached the Kentish Town surgery at 10.40, ten minutes late. Twenty patients waiting. The usual variety— women needing a 'queue tonic', children with skin troubles and coughs, girls sent home from work with 'flu, men with sciatica and lumbago, a young man with acne and a young woman with TB, asking if she could have eggs (the answer had to be "No"). In between looking at tongues, taking temperatures and chatting cheerfully, the doctor filled in forms and cards and made up most of his own prescriptions. "Ridiculous for a doctor to be wasting time like this," he grumbled as he made up a sticky ointment on a slab. It was his only grumble of the day.

There were nine telephone calls. He made three himself, ordering a vaccination outfit, new stocks of drugs, and arranging for a businessman going to the East to have anti-plague and yellow fever injections. At 11.35 we were in the car again, the doctor never missing a move in the traffic game, for more visits. We came to a cottage in a cul-de-sac where the mother of eight children was in bed with rheumatism. He had brought six of them into the world, and the three under five were there to greet him as well as the sixteen-year-old daughter, who was staying home from work to take her mother's place.

"You're a wonderful woman," the doctor said. "With all you do, it's a marvel you keep your feet at all. Two more days in bed and the same treatment and you won't die yet awhile."

Then he gave some instructions and guidance to the 'deputy mother' in the kitchen, and we were waved off enthusiastically at 11.55. More traffic-dodging and three more patients visited. One of them had baked him a cake. That reminded him to stop at a bakery and pick up the family bread. "My surgery towels are all in rags. Must try to get coupons for some new ones."

We lunched near his West End consulting-room with his wife. ("I like seeing her now and then!") She had half a dozen messages for him. "How's the time?", he asked as the coffee came in at two.

All the patients at his consulting-room were rheumatic. They got five or ten minutes each—thirteen patients in ninety minutes. Rheumatism is the doctor's speciality, and

his secret hope is to devote himself to it one day. He has no
time to give his patients treatment himself, so he sends
them to clinics or physiotherapists.

At 3.45 we started for his Highgate surgery, for the first of
eight patients, who got about ten minutes each.

Then, at 5.30, came his first peaceful interval of the day—
high tea at home. Over his second cup he became unexpectedly personal. "I live on a strict diet. I've given up smoking.
Have a tendency to duodenal ulcer. I suppose I work from
eleven to thirteen hours a day. I dread the winter. Frankly, I
don't think I can stand the pace much longer. I used to love
my work. Now I'm getting an active dislike of it. Why?
Because I'm obliged to skimp it. Not good for anybody, least
of all a doctor. Besides, there's no time for research and
reading. Let me tell you one thing—demobbing of doctors
can't be too soon. How's the time?"

I had thought his day's work done. Not at all. There were
twenty-five patients waiting for him at the Kentish Town
surgery. He was there at 6.5, only five minutes late. I sat
with the patients, who seemed to regard waiting as a social
occasion. "Doctor has a hard life, and does his best," they
agreed. When the last one left, I joined the doctor in his
dispensary. He was bent over a test-tube as it bubbled in a
gas flame.

"How's the time?" he asked. We both laughed our first
laugh of the day. It was 8.30, and he had forgotten he had
half a dozen specimens to analyse. It would be nine before
the ordinary, routine, thirteen-hour day of a post-war GP
was done.

It was this heavy burden of responsibility and workload
which I hoped the Health Centres would relieve, thus
helping to make us all better doctors. Whether this would
have developed, we shall never know. I doubt there were
even ten Health Centres ten years later and certainly none
which compared with the blueprint which my committee
had published. If they had been set up in any numbers,
there must have been many doctors, like myself, who
would have helped to air and discuss so many of the
problems of diagnosis and treatment which have been
described in this book. If that had happened, then maybe
we should not have had to endure all these long, fruitless
years. Recommendations from a group of thinking doctors

in Health Centres could not have been ignored in the same way as my own effort. Without this type of discussion, the old order will not change, either in its thinking or in its habits.

10

The Stifling of New Ideas

I am fairly sure that all of you who have read so far will
wonder why, if all I have said is true, the medical profession
did not read my book and welcome its new approach. Surely
the profession would gladly seize on any new idea which
offered even the faintest hope of a solution to some of its
problems! The assumption was proved wrong, and I should
have known it, because of (a) my experience with the
Migraine Trust and (b) the long list of doctors who in the past
failed to get their ideas accepted by the medical profession.

First, let me tell you the story of the effort I made some
three years ago, when I approached the Migraine Trust. I
spent some time with the Medical Director explaining in
detail what the theory and practice of my treatment were. I
offered to treat a selected number of patients under their
supervision and participation, in order to establish whether
there was any real truth in my claim. What I particularly
wanted to find out was how often a rheumatic patch could
be found in an unselected number of established migraine
cases, and whether I could achieve results similar to those I
had treated. I further made it quite clear that it would not
cost the Trust a single penny. I was prepared to provide all
the necessary materials at my own expense. She seemed

quite genuinely interested and suggested I send in an immediate application. She did not want me to miss the Advisory Council's next meeting some three days later as there would not be another for at least a month. I honestly believe she was as keen as I was to start the investigation. You can now see my application dated 18th November. On 25th November the Council secretary wrote to tell me that my application had been rejected by the council and no reason given.

APPLICATION TO CLINIC MANAGEMENT COMMITTEE
18th November 1974

I do not request a grant of any kind. All I require is the facility to examine, and treat where appropriate, about twenty to thirty patients. This number should be sufficient to establish whether there is a clinically demonstrable chronic rheumatic factor which might respond to treatment. Successful treatment would become obvious in a matter of weeks.

As pointed out to Dr Wilkinson in a personal interview, I have treated two patients with long histories of migraine. One has remained free for five years and the other for one year, without taking any drugs whatever.

I am aware that two cases is very minute. That is why I wish to pursue the investigation.

I then wrote the following letter to Dr Wilkinson:

27th November 1974

Dear Dr Wilkinson:

I was naturally disappointed that your Medical Advisory Council did not feel able to afford me facilities for my research.

As you know, I disclosed to you at our interview the details of my past research and the method I proposed to adopt in treating selected cases of migraine.

I would, therefore, be glad if you would be good enough to send me a letter confirming that I have given you this information.

Yours sincerely,
William W. Fox

Dr Marcia Wilkinson MA DM FRCP
The Princess Margaret Migraine Clinic

I received a most gracious reply from her in which she repeated her interest in my views and her regret that my application was turned down.

I wonder whether you would agree with the Advisory Council's curt attitude to another member of the profession. I do understand why, and maybe you do now. In Chapter II I explained the inability of the specialist mind to give credence to anything not explicable in known disease patterns. Was I not entitled to a reasoned statement as to why they refused an offer which would cost them nothing and which might add some knew knowledge to what is, in effect, an incomprehensible disease?

The book was submitted to three publishers, who each took about seven weeks to reject it. My agent assured me that this was quite usual in the trade and could go on for a very long time yet; a dozen refusals was quite on the cards. Rightly or wrongly, I took the view that these refusals were based on the fact that I was not on the staff of a hospital or university and was not well-known, and, therefore, that the book would have less chance of profitable sales. After all, that is what the publishers are in business for—not to promote challenging views from an unprominent doctor. Furthermore, at my age I was not prepared to wait another year or two for their patronage. I resolved to become my own publisher. At least, I was prepared to back my forty years' work with my own money.

There was no difficulty in finding a printer, and within four months the book was ready, with review copies being sent to all the medical journals, national newspapers, magazines, radio, television etc. It was greeted with the most stunning silence since the introduction of the Cenotaph Service. Some time later two ripples disturbed the terribly calm waters of silence. First, London Broadcasting gave me an interview which was broadcast, and then one of the television networks recorded another interview with me about the book. Although I was given a date for its broadcast, they phoned later to cancel the date with an excuse for its delay, which has continued to date. I was surprised and disappointed that no journal or newspaper had thought fit even to notice the book.

However, as time went by, I learned from bitter experience that a privately published book was viewed with suspicion. Why would not any publisher undertake it? The next important lesson I learned was that all the media, with the one exception of London Broadcasting, will not even look at an orthodox medical publication unless it has been accepted by the medical Establishment. This really means that it must emanate from one of the universities, medical schools or hospitals. Failing that, it must have received some form of support in the *British Medical Journal* or the *Lancet*, the only two medical journals which the scientific and medical correspondents of all the media consult. This attitude of the correspondents is not unreasonable, but it does rather stifle their initiative and tends to presuppose that any other member of the medical profession is something of a moron!

After a while I wrote to the *Lancet* to ask if they were going to review my book. They wrote back and said that there were so many books submitted for review, they could not possibly do them all. They regretted that my book was not to be reviewed. I wrote back and asked how they could ignore a book which claimed a new and successful approach in a field of medicine which was bankrupt of any ideas. Was it not part of a medical journal's duty to put forward new ideas? A formal printed acknowledgement put an end to this correspondence.

At the same time I wrote to the *British Medical Journal*. Their reply was most encouraging. Yes, they had sent my book for review by their consultant rheumatologist, and I could expect the review to appear in about six or seven weeks' time. Alas! It did not appear, and I then contacted the Review Editor. He was kindness itself and said that he would make enquiries. He phoned back later and told me that the consultant had refused to review the book. I asked if any reason had been given, and he replied that it was not done to ask for a reason. "Well, could you not ask somebody else to review it?" I asked. The answer, predictably, was that they could not possibly do that. A doctor whom I had treated at that time, and who was very appreciative of my work, wrote to the *British Medical Journal*, telling of her experience with my treatment and urged them not to let my work go unreviewed. They wrote back expressing their interest but regretted they could do no more.

Some 2 years earlier, the late Dr W. S. C. Copeman, who was then the leader of the rheumatologists in Britain and the editor of the BMA publication *Annals of Rheumatism*, personally reviewed an article of mine entitled "A New Approach to the Cause and Medical Treatment of Arthritis of the Hip". In that journal—no small compliment to an outsider like me. This article formed an integral part of my book, and indeed the discovery of the rheumatic patch developed directly from that work.

Prior to this Mr Rodney Maingot, Editor-in-Chief of the *British Journal of Clinical Practice* had published and congratulated me on the excellence of that work. When Mr Maingot read the book, he wrote me a personal note of congratulation and said that the book would be sent for review to a rheumatologist. *World Medicine*, a very excellent commercial publication which I enjoy reading—indeed, I look forward to it each fortnight, also submitted it for review to a rheumatologist. Neither journal was able to get a review.

So there you have it—three unknown (to me) rheumatologists (or maybe they were all the same person, an interesting but unlikely situation) would not review my book.

How can this sort of behaviour on the part of these rheumatologists be explained when one considers the many flattering opinions of my book—opinions expressed and written by a number of doctors who have referred cases to me over many many years?

I am an orthodox medical practitioner who has practised medicine for more years than ever they are likely to do. I have produced results documented in my book which startled me. I was actually able to improve patients by applying methods of treatment based on the deductions made from the detailed clinical study described in the test. There was no other known way by which these people could be helped. None of these successes could be ascribed to natural remission. The results were predicted at the time when the treatment was given, and they happened almost at once. How could any doctor reading these reports presume to ignore them?

I cannot and do not claim to cure everybody. A considerable number can be helped, and all I am saying is "Please look, here is a new approach, a new hope." The cost to investigate it is infinitesimal. More money and effort are wasted in one single day in the NHS than this investigation, with all its promise, could possibly cost. That people are worried about the continuing failure to solve the arthritic problem, there is no doubt. Could that be a reason why, in spite of nil publicity, the demand for my book has reached nearly six hundred copies? Being my own publisher, I know that most of the demand has come, via the public, from libraries all over the country.

To have been thwarted by the medical Establishment is disappointment enough, but I cannot put my pen down until I have told the story of the ultimate stronghold of the medical profession, the General Medical Council. On 10th November 1975, the President of the Council caused a letter to be sent to me in which I was asked to explain some details about an advertisement in *The Times* (also in the *Daily Telegraph* which they did not mention) regarding my book. The fact that these queries were made showed that his advisers, if he had any, did not understand the simple fundamental rights of an author and publisher to advertise his book. Worst of all they referred to some passages in my book in which they accused me of making "invidious" comparisons between the results of my treatment and those of other doctors. Can you conceive of my feelings on receiving this kind of correspondence from them after devoting a lifetime to the study of these dreadful diseases, and then spending my own money in trying to get the ideas across to the profession?

You can now read a copy of my letter in reply which I sent three days later.

13th November 1975

Dear Sir,

I acknowledge the receipt of your letter, and reply to your queries as follows:

1. The treatment is successful, so why should it not be so described? You will find the point dealt with in the final paragraph in the book.

2. I am the publisher of the book and can conduct its business only from a known address. There are other reasons, but this should suffice.

3. I am more than a little surprised at the choice of words "invidious comparisons". It indicates that the reader has failed to appreciate the theme of the book. May I clarify! The book describes in detail an entirely new clinical finding and treatment which, except by a remarkable coincidence, could not be known to any other doctor.

I am not, therefore, criticizing or denigrating any member of the profession but merely demonstrating that, with this new knowledge, it is feasible to achieve results after correct diagnosis and assessment, which hitherto were not thought possible. (Please read Case XVI with comments.)

Can you suggest any other way in which these claims can be substantiated, except by treating proven failed cases and improving them? These are the cases that seek my aid.

In the context of your letter, it is well for you to know that I am seventy years of age, with angina, and not, therefore, seeking either patients or preferment. I simply want the profession to test my claims and not unnecessarily delay the relief it can afford to countless sufferers.

As the book has been looked at with ethical points in mind, I would suggest it be read as I intended, for its moral, clinical and therapeutic values.

I am enclosing a copy of the letter sent with the book to the medical journals. It sums up my attitude.

Yours faithfully,
William W. Fox

Dear Sir,

In submitting this book for review by your Journal, may I be permitted to make the following observations.

As you know, there is no real understanding of the pathological process as it affects the various forms of chronic rheumatic disease—there is no correlation between the different types of arthritis and fibrositis and no form of treatment that remotely resembles a cure.

This book is the result of forty years' continuous, clinical study punctuated by a paper presented in 1940 and a second one in 1965, so that in 1975 one can hardly be accused of rushing into print.

In it you will find a new approach to the problem; all the signs, symptoms and histories have been marshalled to give a coherent picture of the disease-processes in the different forms of arthritis. The common factors then become reasonably obvious, particularly when response to treatment based on these findings gives uniformly good results.

Some of these results are so astonishing that an onlooker might be forgiven if he doubted them. In view of the recurring disappointments in research, drug treatment and physical medicine, I can understand this scepticism, which should be dissipated with the study of the cases presented.

The final chapter refers to undiagnosed clinical syndromes which often have the same pathological background. This extra knowledge can eliminate the need for exhaustive and fruitless investigations, whilst adding an extra and positive dimension to differential diagnosis.

Very serious thought has been given to the responsibility of publishing this book, because in dealing with such a widespread disease, we must all be aware that, in the end, we are treating human beings whose hopes and disappointments must be the paramount consideration.

Yours faithfully,
William W. Fox

How groundless were the original charges or queries—I don't mind what you may call them—can be judged from the fact that two months later on 14th January 1976 the secretary sent me a three line letter saying that the President had noted my observations! No apology or retraction of the allegations. You may be quite sure that if I had done anything wrong I would most certainly have been warned, admonished or censured.

A consideration of what this correspondence implies may help you to understand the thinking which pervades the medical Establishment as typified in this case by the President of the General Medical Council and his advisers. I must presume that they read my book with the greatest of care, because being such a powerful body they would be very conscious indeed of their great responsibility not to make allegations which did not have some reasonable basis in fact. The letter demonstrates quite clearly a total inability to distinguish between the presentation of entirely new clinical knowledge, which should have been welcomed, and a supposed criticism of medical inefficiency, which cannot possibly be construed by any rational reading of my book. Such an 'error of judgment' can be ascribed to the minds of people who are so confident and sure of themselves that they cannot conceive of any possible shortcomings in their achievements.

How can one expect the leaders of the profession, who have enjoyed the flattery of success in a limited field, to measure the failure of the profession as a whole to understand and deal with the limitless mass of ill health and consequent unhappiness?

Perhaps it is their subconscious desire to stifle this possibility which led them into a false judgement. The error of judgement in my case must now be crystal clear. How many more may there be which never see the light of day? There are a small number due to inefficiency of individual doctors or the organization, for which there is appropriate machinery, including the General Medical Council and the vigilance of the Patients' Association. The vast numbers, about which I am concerned, are due to a lack of knowledge. There is no guilt in not knowing but there must be in not trying to understand that which is clearly comprehensible and capable of investigation and evaluation.

The whole sad affair left me speechless. However, the utter ungraciousness of the reply, instead of making me angry, stimulated my sense of humour. I turned to my wife and said, "I can only hope that the President who 'noted' my observations is a good musician. Who knows, it might get into the 'charts'—but probably only temperature charts!"

In view of this appalling correspondence, I must make my views absolutely clear. I am not attacking or denigrating any doctor in this country, or indeed in the whole wide world. Whatever they think or do is based on the accepted knowledge and behaviour of the profession. It is the logical and direct result of the method of medical education, which follows the same pattern in probably every country in the world.

Because every effort I have made to be heard by the profession so far has failed, I have written this book for the public. I hope that it has demonstrated that there is much room for self-criticism by the medical profession. If they put their own house in order, they may yet achieve a degree of success in diagnosis and treatment which would make much of the present NHS redundant.

Instead of worrying about whether to sustain life for a few more days or weeks in a patient with a fatal illness, they should be paying far more attention to those people who have to endure endless years of suffering and pain. How can you compare the maintenance of life for a few weeks in a terminal illness to the curing of a young person with arthritis in the hands or feet. May I repeat what I said earlier in the book and which has been one of my guiding tenets: the quality of the life we live is far more important than the length of the life we may have to endure. Because I have always cared about people, I have tried to put disease in its proper place and not to elevate it above mankind.

Epilogue

For at least two years before deciding to write this book, I experienced a sadness tinged with despair that my first book was not able to penetrate the incalculable thickness of the mental wall erected by the rheumatological establishment and their influence on the media. This influence is very real, as I discovered through my contacts with medical and scientific correspondents. They occasionally nibbled at my ideas, but sooner or later enthusiasm waned, perhaps because their comfortable relations with the Establishment, from which they got all the latest medical news, might be disturbed. I certainly understood this wariness, because they must have found it difficult to believe that an independent doctor could know more than the 'experts', for if he did, these experts would surely have afforded him some recognition.

The sadness was not one of self-pity but related to my deep-felt concern for the suffering of all those people who could be helped in the same way as my own patients.

The despair was only a tinge because, in spite of so many rebuffs, I knew I could never resist the persistent urge to make this knowledge generally available, no matter how long it took. This resolution was at last rewarded in 1978 when Dr Freed was sufficiently impressed with my book to invite me to make an audio-visual recording of the essential points in the diagnosis and treatment of the rheumatic patch. This was done at the University of Manchester in November 1979. It was after this and through his good offices that research on the rheumatic patch for a possible virus was undertaken by Dr D. A. J. Tyrrell at The Clinical Research Centre, Northwick Park. Further investigations on the allergic aspect of these patches is being carried at Manchester University. These activities, together with the confirmation of the value of the diphtheroid treatment carried out independently in France, have underlined three of the most important aspects of the rheumatic disease which I first wrote about in 1950.

So why can I not rest content and wait for further developments?

Well, if you have not guessed by now, then I have to say that I will be seventy-five when you are reading this book, and cannot therefore wait too long—certainly not another thirty years—to reach my objectives. They are, firstly, that everybody who can benefit from this treatment should be able to get it without delay. It requires no expensive paraphernalia; treatments take relatively little time, and the cost is infinitesimal. The second is that the principles of diagnosis and treatment, based on orthodox clinical evidence which I have collected over all these years, should be made available to the whole of the medical profession and its students. This would help to make diagnosis of both rheumatic and allied conditions more precise, whilst the inevitable analysis and criticism from its practitioners should help to refine its values, for there is surely much more to be studied before a total cure is achieved.

Everything I have learned about the rheumatic and allied conditions has come from the collective wisdom of all those patients to whom I listened over the years. I have now organized this knowledge and present it back to you, in gratitude for the indescribable happiness it gave me when I was able to give real help in restoring function and reducing pain without drugs.

Use this knowledge to pressurize those entrenched and

misguided members of the medical profession, few in number but powerful in their position, who block progress simply because they live in mental splints and not because they are any less well-intentioned than any other doctor.

No doctor wants a patient to suffer, so see to it that they know as much as you now do.

meraus.

colibris